Thank you very much for choosing my low-carb recipe book for a week. After reviewing it, please give me a review with the content of what you liked and / or did not like. Your review is very important to me to make my following books more sophisticated for you. I thank you in advance for taking the time for your review.

Table of contents

The low-carb nutrition plan

A low-carbohydrate diet can help you lose weight. I have put together a low-carb nutrition plan here that provides a selection of delicious low-carb meals for a whole week.

Basics of the nutrition plan according to Low-Carb

With the low-carb diet plan, the intake of carbohydrates is drastically reduced - protein- and fat-rich foods, however, are allowed almost indefinitely. This is intended to ensure that the body obtains its energy predominantly from fats and protein instead of carbohydrates.

The dishes in this low-carb nutrition plan are suitable for satiety, so you can eat a little more than the usual portion.

This form of nutrition does not focus on a calorie-reduced diet, but on a protein-rich diet.

This means that the low-carb nutrition plan can be individually adapted to your personal energy requirements and supplemented with other foods in the sense of low-carb nutrition.

Day 1 Breakfast

Vegetable omelette with tomatoes and peppers

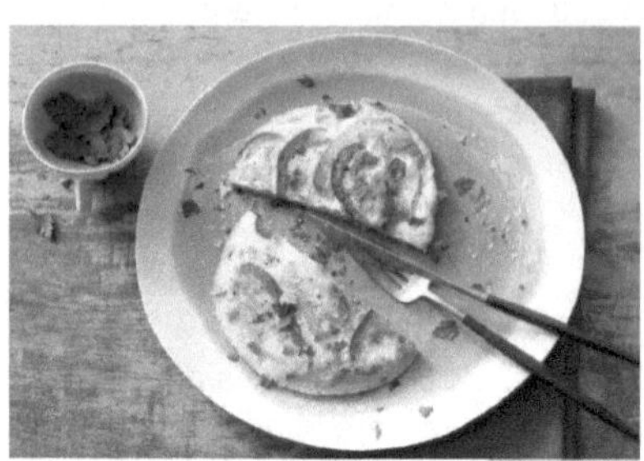

The low-carb nutrition plan starts with a vegetable omelette with tomatoes and peppers (200 calories per serving) for breakfast. The quick pan dish delivers high-quality protein that is satiating for a long time and does not allow for ravenous appetite attacks. Peppers provide vitamin C and bite in the meal!

<u>Difficulty</u>:   easy
<u>Preparation</u>:   25 minutes
<u>Calories</u>:   200 kcal

Ingredients for 2 + portions

1 onion 250 g
small peppers (1 red, 1 yellow, 2 small peppers)
160 g tomatoes (2 tomatoes)
1 sprig of thyme
1 garlic clove
1 tablespoon of olive oil
2 eggs
40 g sour cream (2 tablespoons)
salt, pepper, nutmeg
6 stems flat parsley

Preparation

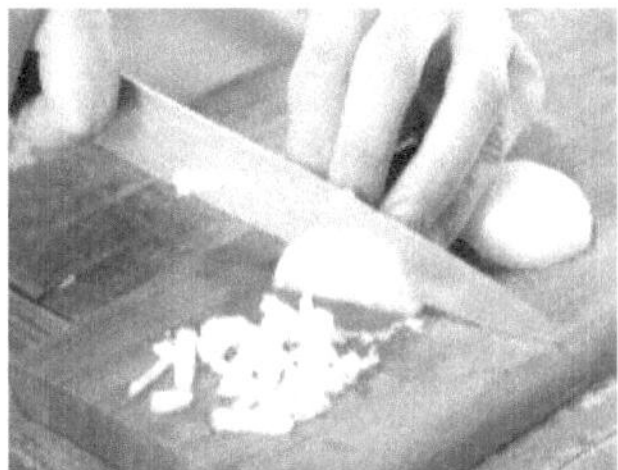

Peel and chop the onion.

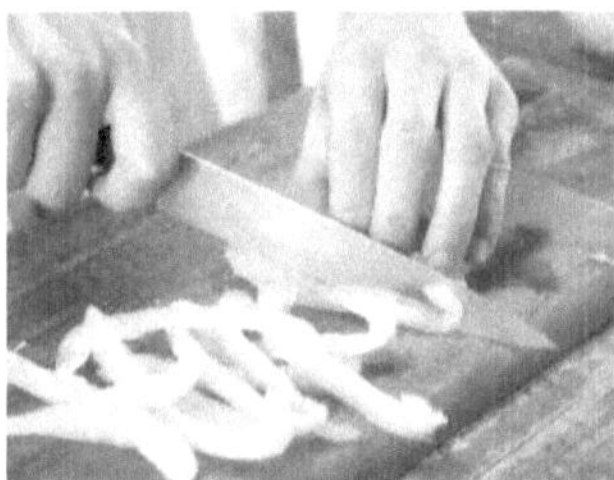

Halve the peppers, remove seeds, wash and cut into fine strips.

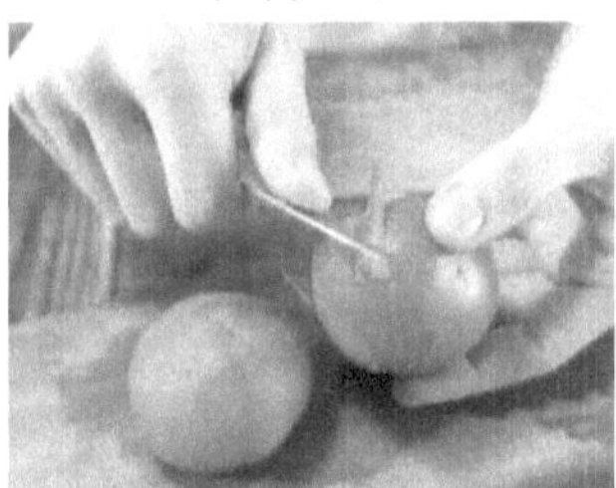

Cut out the stems of the tomatoes in a wedge shape. Dip the tomatoes briefly in boiling water, remove, rinse cold and remove the skin. Dice the tomatoes.

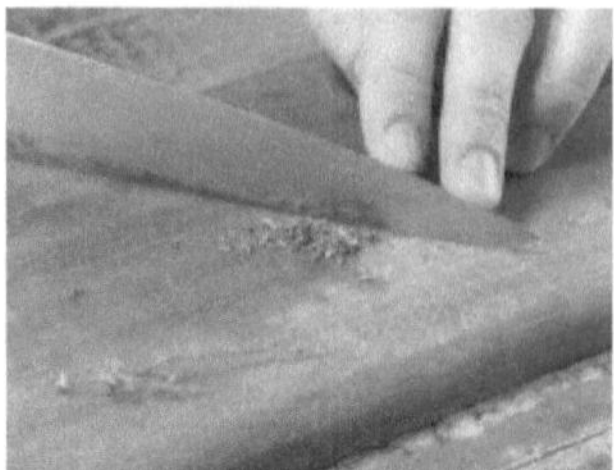

Thyme wash, shake dry, pluck off leaves and chop finely.

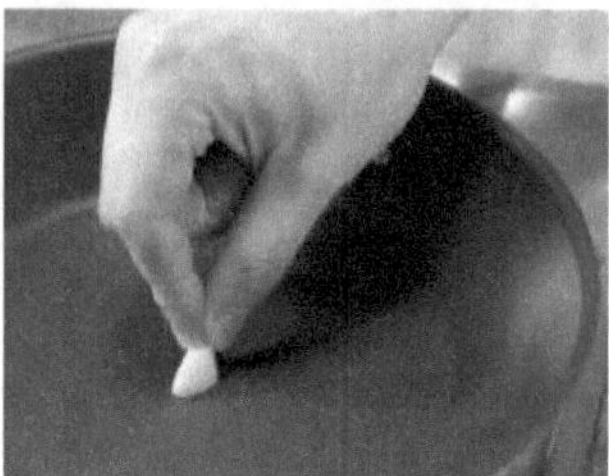

Peel and halve the garlic. Rub a coated pan with the halved clove of garlic.

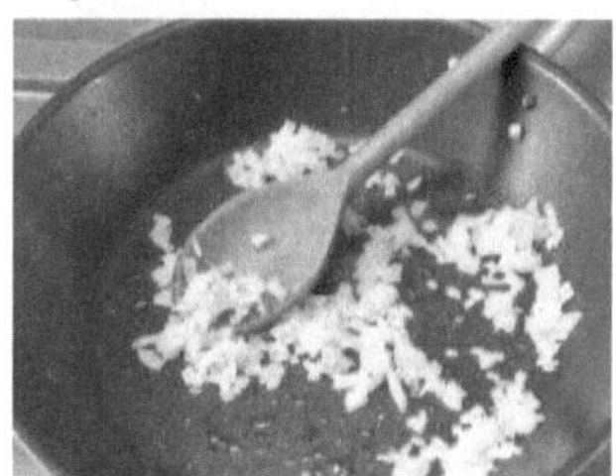

Heat the oil in the pan. Sauté the onion cubes and thyme over medium heat.

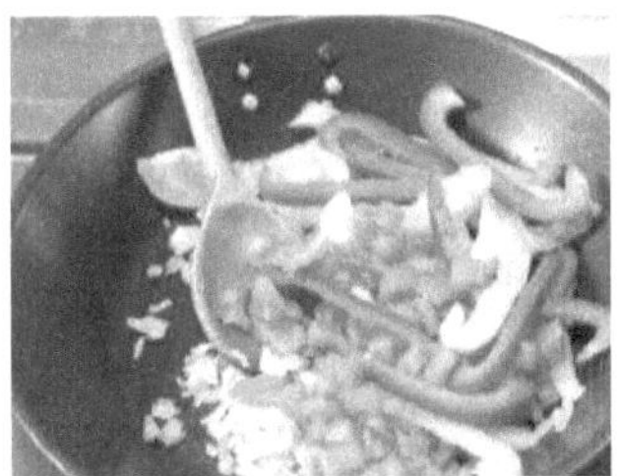

Add pepper strips and steam for 2-3 minutes, add diced tomatoes and steam for another 2-3 minutes.

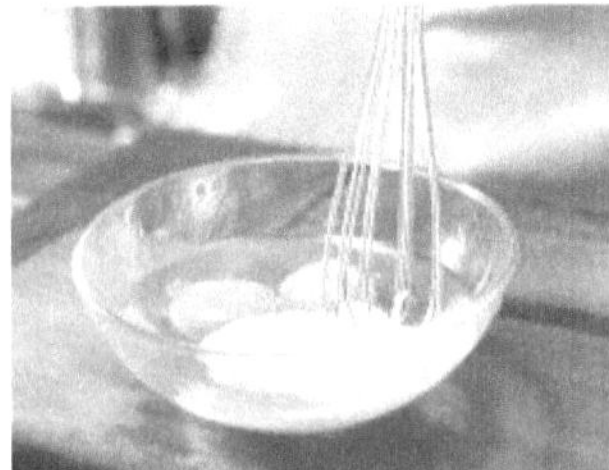

Whisk eggs and sour cream, season with salt, pepper and grated nutmeg. Pour the egg mixture over the vegetables and let it simmer at low heat for 5-8 minutes (depending on how firm you like the egg).

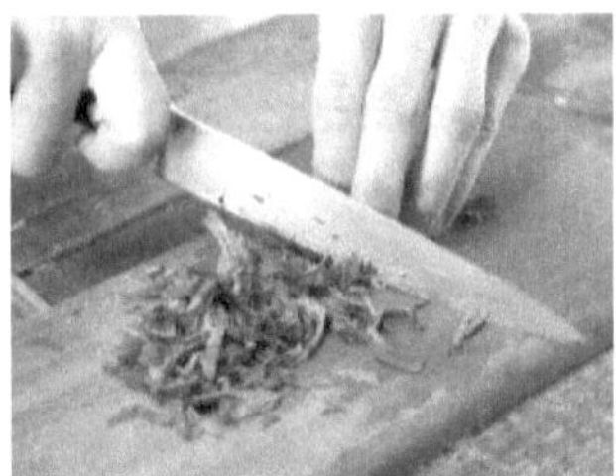

Wash parsley, shake dry, pluck off leaves and chop. Sprinkle on the vegetable omelette and serve.

Nutritional values

1 Portion contains	(percentage of the daily	requirement)
Calories	200 kcal	(10 %)
Protein	10 g	(10 %)
fat	14 g	(12 %)
Carbohydrates	8 g	(5 %)
added sugar	0 g	(0 %)
Fibres	5,5 g	(18 %)

This recipe is healthy because...

The ingredients can hardly deny that this is a variation of the
original Basque name, called "Piperade". They don't have to,
because our version tastes just as delicious - but it gets by with
much less fat.

Day 1 Snack
filled mini cucumber with tomato cream cheese

As a delicious snack for in-between, there is this low-carb meal: filled
mini cucumber with tomato cream cheese (100 calories per portion).
The low-carb grainy cream cheese is one of the best foods in a low-
carb diet, as it also contains a lot of satiating protein.

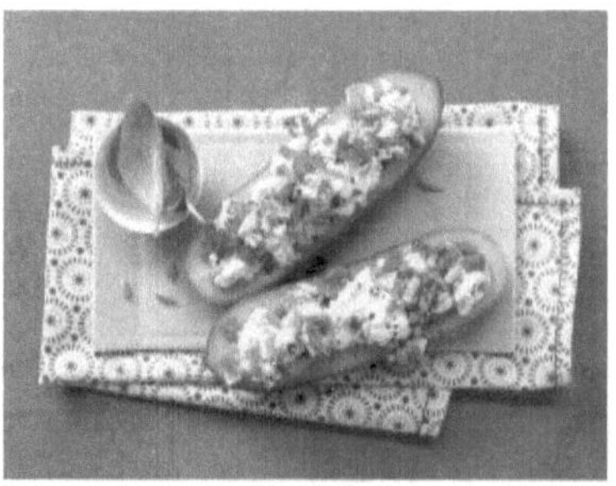

Ingredients for 1+ portion

1 Mini Cucumber
1 tsp. Sunflower seeds
3 cherry tomatoes
75 g granular cream cheese (0,8 % fat)
Salt
Pepper
2 basil stems

Difficulty: very simple
Preparation: 15 Minutes
Calories: 100 kcal

Preparation

Wash the cucumber, rub dry, cut in half lengthwise and

remove seeds with a teaspoon.

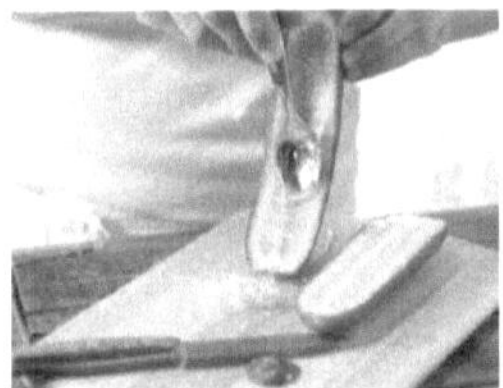

Roast sunflower seeds in a coated pan without fat until light brown.

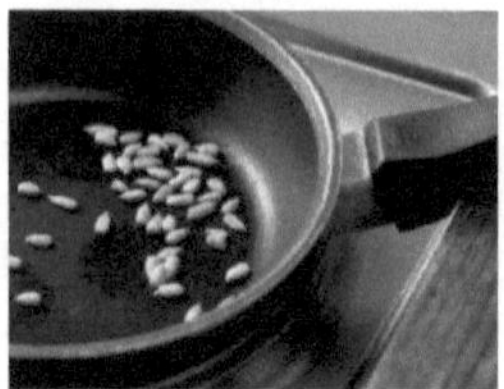

Wash and quarter the tomatoes, cut out the stalk and dice the flesh.

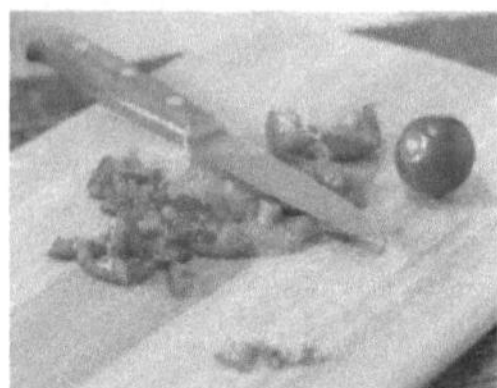

Mix cream cheese in a small bowl with sunflower seeds and tomato cubes. Season to taste with salt and pepper.

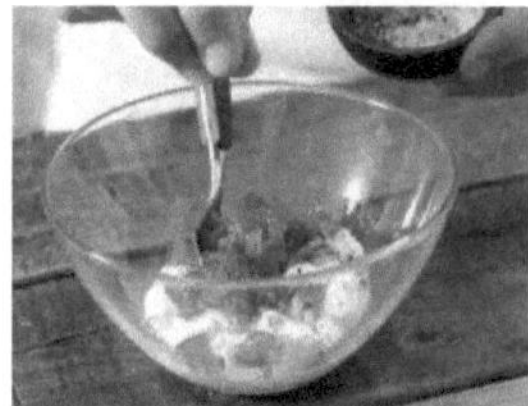

Wash basil, shake dry, pluck leaves and cut into fine strips. Fill the tomato cream cheese into the cucumber halves, sprinkle with basil and serve.

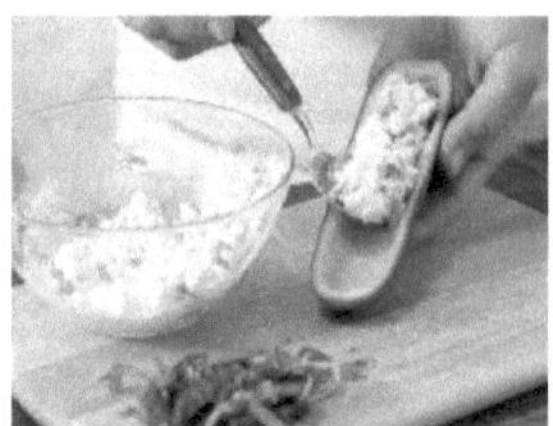

Nutritional values

1 Portion contains	(percentage of daily	requirement)
Calories	100 kcal	(5 %)
Protein	12 g	(12 %)
Fat	3 g	(3 %)
Carbohydrates	5 g	(3 %)
added sugar	0 g	(0 %)
Fibres	1 g	(3 %)

This recipe is healthy because...

The particularly low content of saturated fatty acids in this
generally very low-fat, fresh vegetable meal is particularly
pleasing to all those who suffer from fat metabolism disorders,
diabetes and high blood pressure. Because here they can enjoy it
without hesitation!
If the amount of carbohydrates ingested is less than 100 grams per
day, this is known as a low-carb diet. Especially in the evening, it is
important to eat a low-carb diet, as this way the fat burning
process is not blocked overnight.

Day 1 Lunch

Italian escalope chasseur

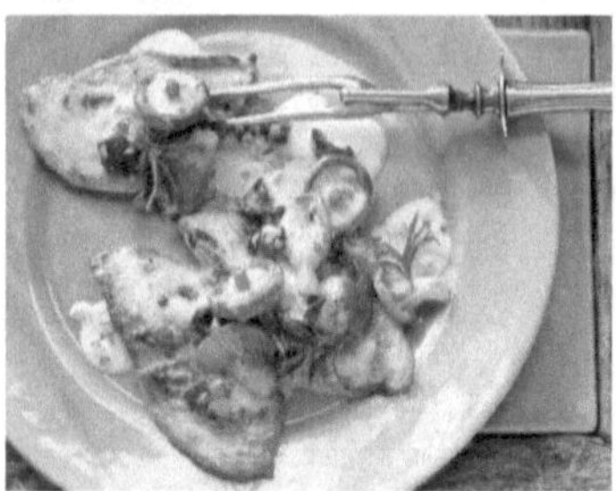

Italian Escalope chausseur (358 calories per serving) makes lunch a delicious affair in the low-carb diet. It is on the table in just 30 minutes and tastes wonderfully Mediterranean. Oyster mushrooms and shiitake mushrooms are low in calories, satisfy well and provide vitamin D compared to other foods.

Difficulty: easy
Preparation: 30 Minutes
Calories: 358 kcal

Ingredients für 4 + portions

250 g small oyster mushrooms
250 g Shiitake mushrooms
2 shallots
50 g dried tomato in oil
1 sprig of rosemary
12 thin chicken breast escalopes à 40 g
3 tablespoons of olive oil
Salt
250 ml soy cream
150 ml dark veal stock

Preparation

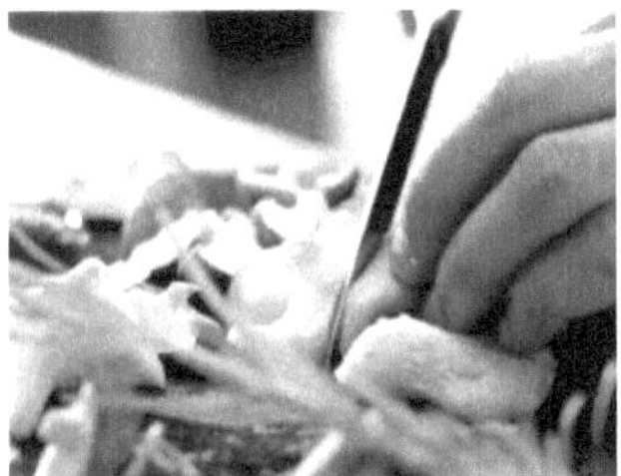

Cleaning mushrooms. Halve oyster mushrooms if necessary.

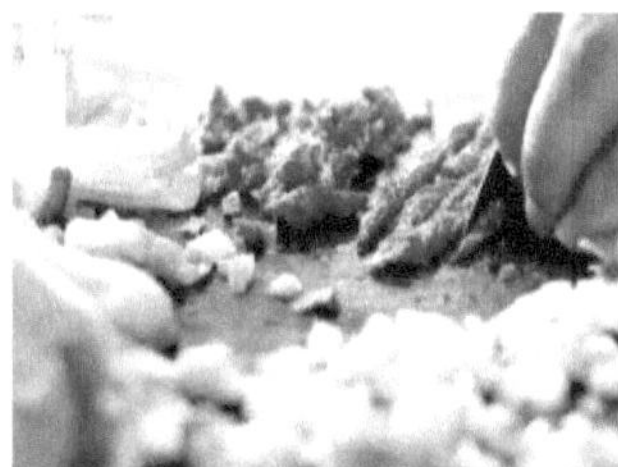

Peel and finely dice the shallots. Cut tomatoes into fine cubes.

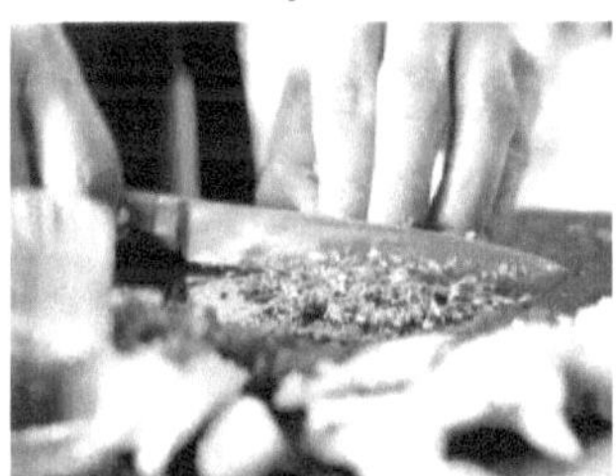

Wash rosemary, shake dry, pluck needles and chop.

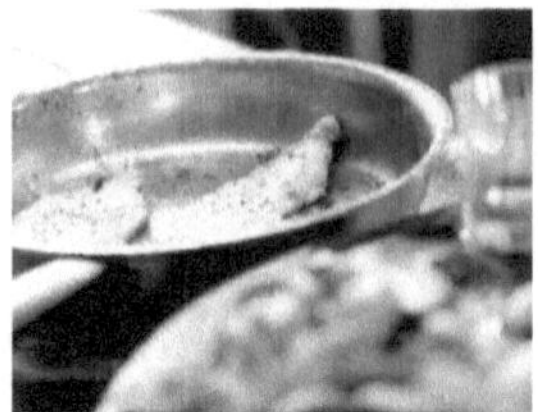

Wash the Escalope and dab dry. Heat 2 tablespoons of oil in a frying pan and fry the escalopes in it over high heat on each side for about 20 seconds.

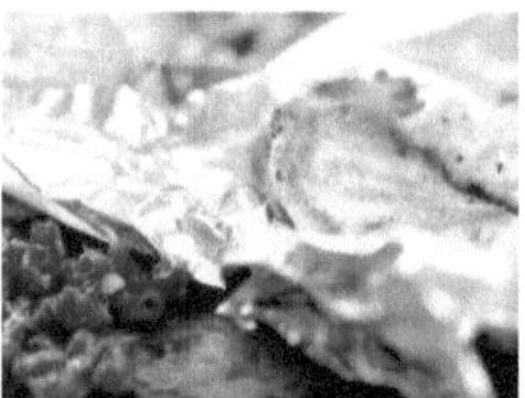

Remove the escalopes from the pan, salt them and keep them warm wrapped up.

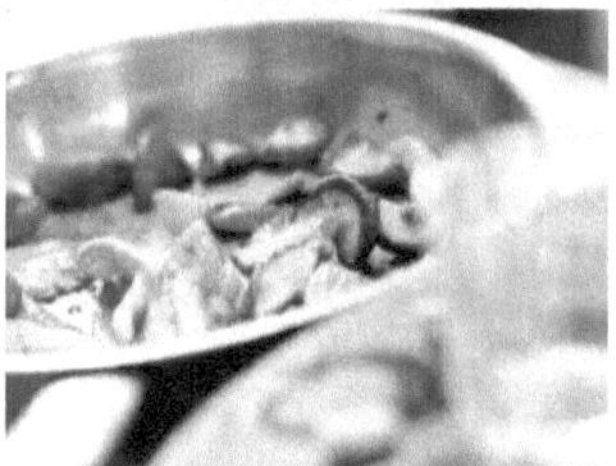

Pour the remaining oil into the pan and fry the mushrooms in it over a high heat for 1 minute while stirring.

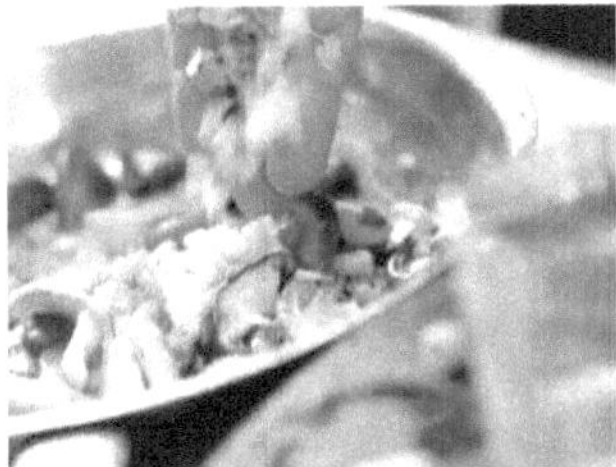

Add the shallots and fry for 1 more minute at medium heat.

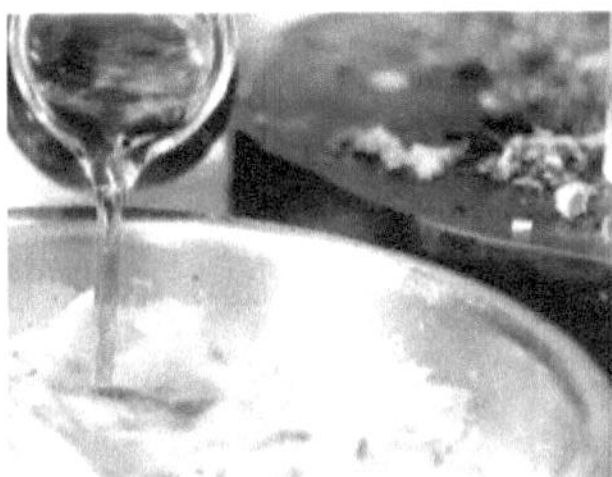

Add the soy cream and veal stock.

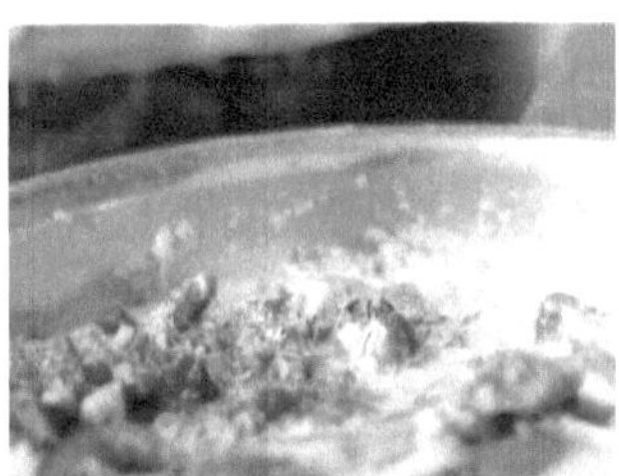

Add dried tomatoes and rosemary. Let everything boil down at low heat for a few minutes until the sauce becomes creamy.

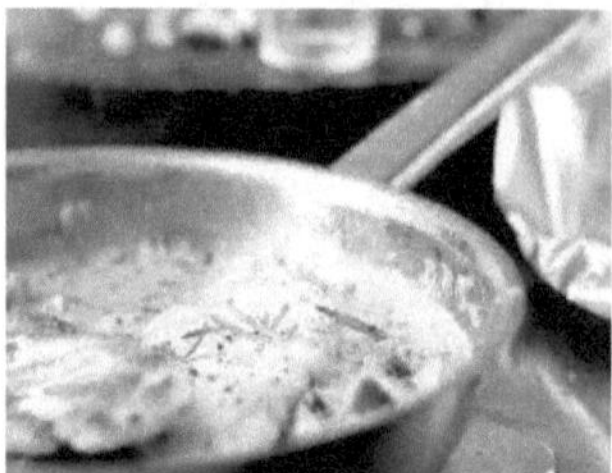

Add the Escalope to the sauce and warm up briefly. Arrange cutlets on plates and serve with the mushroom sauce. Natural rice goes well with it.

This recipe is healthy because...

Oyster mushrooms and shiitake mushrooms are very filling and low in calories. Compared to other vegetable foods, they provide a good portion of vitamin D, which strengthens our immune system and our bones.

Nutritional values

1 Portion contains	(percentage of daily	requirement)
Calories	358 kcal	(17 %)
Protein	34 g	(35 %)
Fat	19 g	(16 %)
Carbohydrates	12 g	(8 %)
added sugar	0 g	(0 %)
Fibres	4,5 g	(15%)

Day 1 Evening meal

The zucchini carpaccio with basil ricotta dumplings

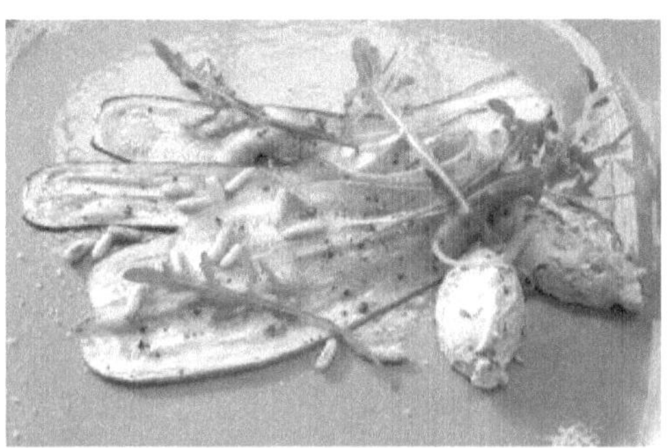

Italian classic as a vegetable version: the zucchini Carpaccio with
basil ricotta dumplings (196 calories per portion) not only tastes
deliciously light, but also covers the daily requirement of biotin. It
supports the formation of creatine, which is important for hair
growth, for example.

Ingredients For 4 portions

300 g small green zucchini (2 small green zucchini)
150 g yellow small zucchini (1 yellow small zucchini)
3 tablespoons of olive oil
Salt
Pepper
30 g pickled dried tomatoes
30 g green olives (without stone)
½ bunch Basil
175 g Ricotta
1 dried chili pepper
20 g Pine nuts

Preparation

Wash one zucchini and cut off the ends. Cut them lengthwise into 5 mm thin slices with a vegetable slicer.

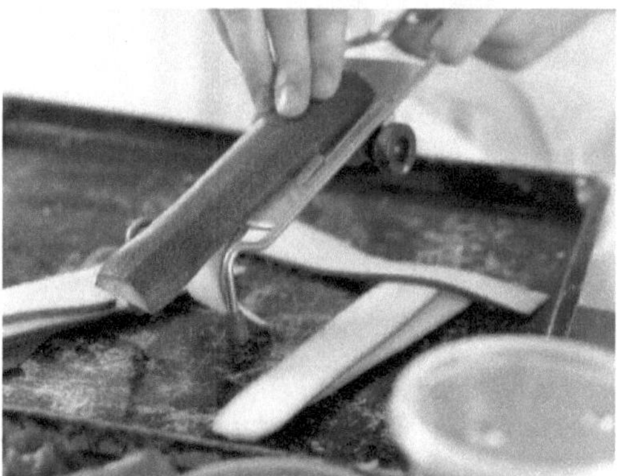

Put zucchini slices on a baking tray, brush with a little oil and season with salt and pepper. Bake in a preheated oven at 220 °C (fan oven 200 °C, gas: level 3-4) on the middle shelf for 8 minutes. Remove and let cool.

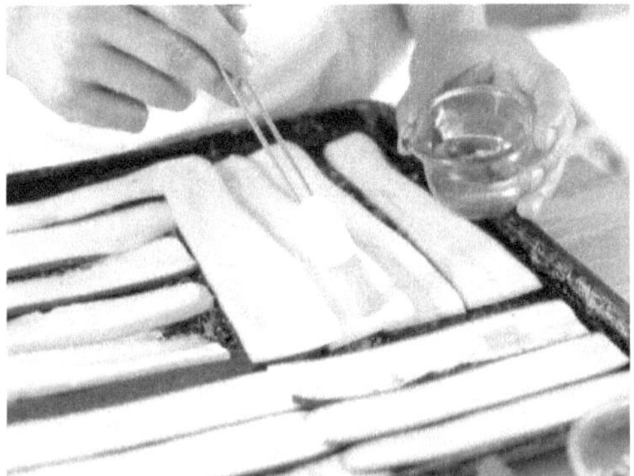

Drain the dried tomatoes. Finely chop the olives. Wash basil, shake dry, pluck off leaves and chop finely. Chop drained tomatoes very finely.

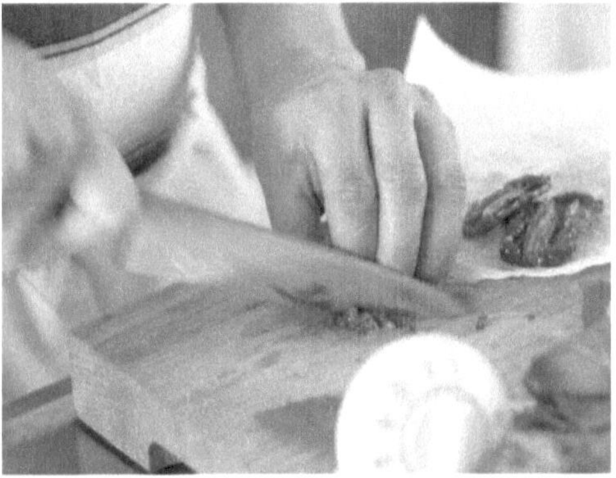

Mix tomatoes, olives and basil with ricotta in a bowl, season with salt, pepper and some crumbled chili pepper.

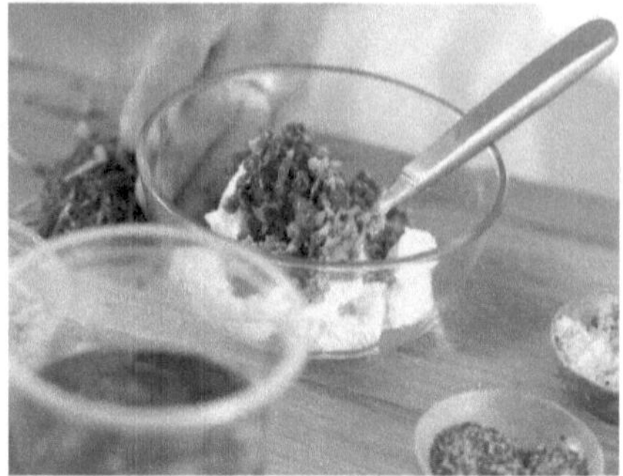

Roast pine nuts in a pan without fat. Clean, wash and spin
dry the rocket.

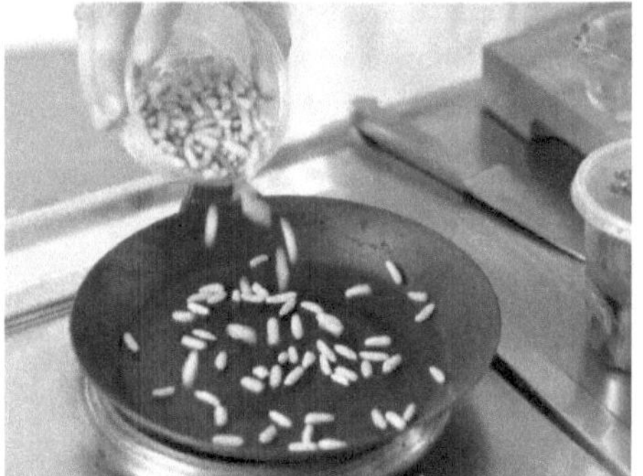

Put zucchini slices on plates. Add 2 moistened
Take tablespoons of the ricotta mixture, cut off the cams and add them
to the zucchini on the plates. Garnish with pine nuts and rocket.

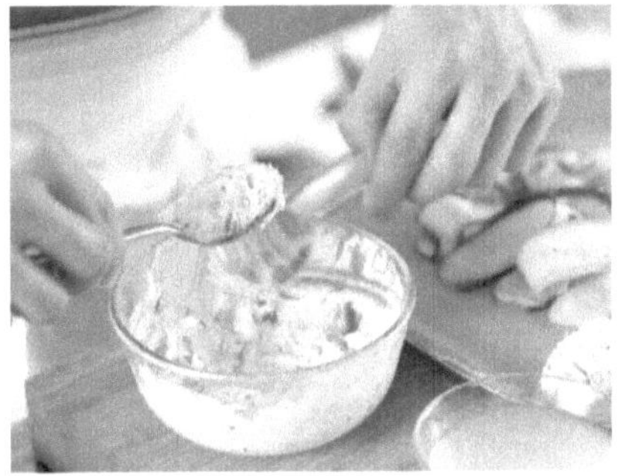

Nutritional values

1 Portion contains	(percentage of daily	requirement)
Calories	196 kcal	(10 %)
Protein	9 g	(18 %)
Fat	15 g	(19 %)
Carbohydrates	6 g	(2 %)
added sugar	0 g	(0 %)
Fibres	3 g	(10 %)

Day 2 Breakfast: Mozzarella with olives and dried tomatoes

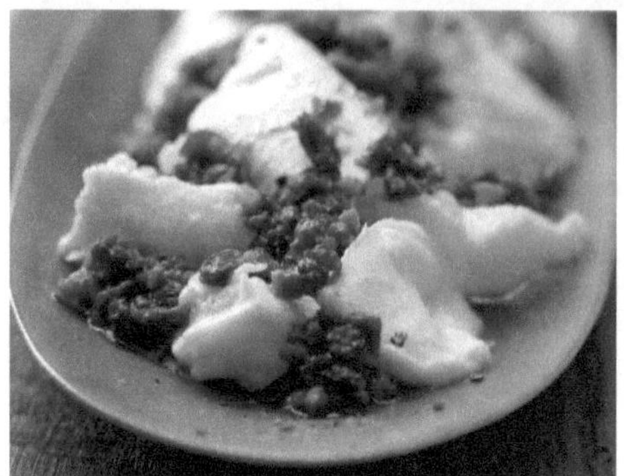

With marinated mozzarella with olives and dried tomatoes (183 calories
per serving), Tuesday morning starts in the low-carb diet. The olive oil
processed in it contains plenty of oleic acid. This belongs to the
monounsaturated fatty acids and helps, among other things, to reduce
inflammatory processes in the blood vessels.

Difficulty: easy
Preparation: 10 minutes
Calories: 183 kcal

Ingredients for 4 portions

½ Lime
40 g green olives without stone
50 g dried tomatoes (drained)
2 tablespoons of olive oil
1 small dried chili pepper
250 g mozzarella (9 % fat)
black pepper rosemary to garnish

Preparation

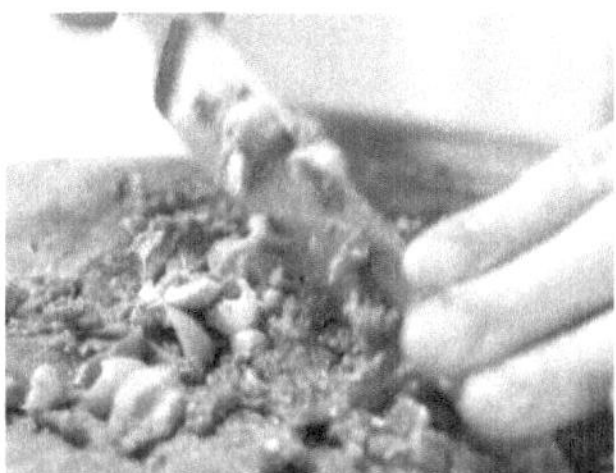

Squeeze the lime, measure 1 tablespoon of juice. Finely chop
the olives and dried tomatoes.

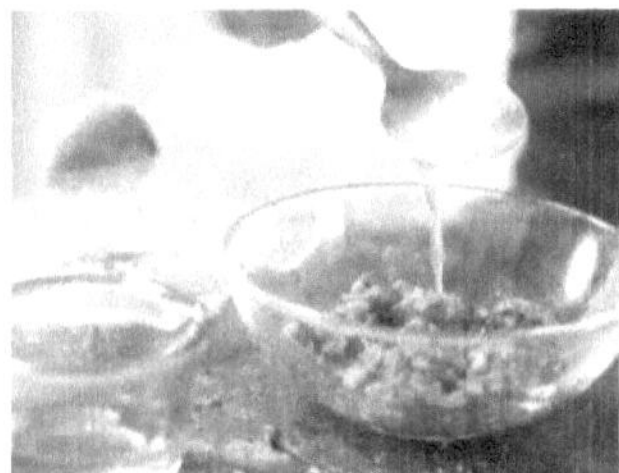

Drain the cheese and cut into small pieces.

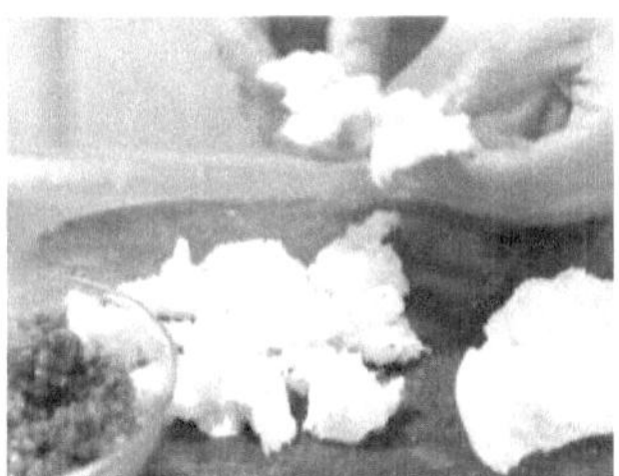

Put the cheese on a plate and season with pepper. With the
Sprinkle the seasoning oil and leave to stand (marinate) at room
temperature for 15 minutes. Serve garnished with some rosemary.

This recipe is healthy because...

Olives and their oil contain a lot of oleic acid, a monounsaturated
fatty acid. Thus they improve the ratio between "good" and "bad"
cholesterol, lower blood pressure and slow down inflammatory
processes in the blood vessels. Especially people with a high risk of
cardiovascular diseases benefit from this.

Nutritional values

1 Portion contains	(percentage of daily	requirement)
Calories	183 kcal	(9 %)
Protein	14 g	(14 %)
Fat	12 g	(10 %)
Carbohydrates	4 g	(3 %)
added sugar	0 g	(0 %)
Fibres	0,5 g	(2 %)

Day 2 Snack

Turkey meatballs with paprika

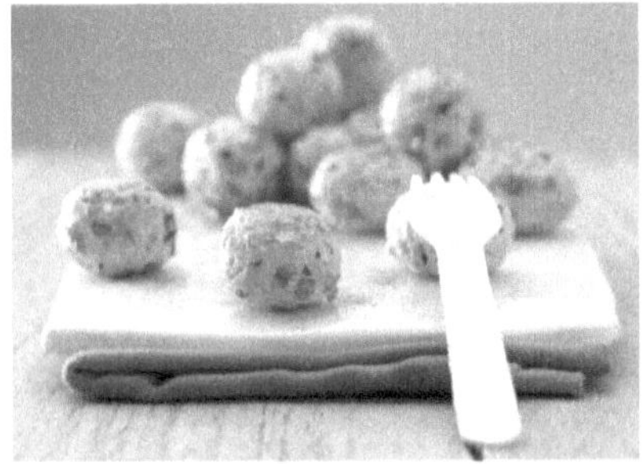

Difficulty: medium
Preparation: 25 minutes
Calories: 160 kcal

Ingredients for - 4 + portions

200 g red pepper (1 red pepper)
40 g onions (1 onion)
1 garlic clove
6 stems of parsley
400 g minced turkey
2 tsp breadcrumbs
3 tablespoons low-fat curd cheese
Salt
Pepper
Cayenne pepper
1 tablespoon rapeseed oil

Preparation

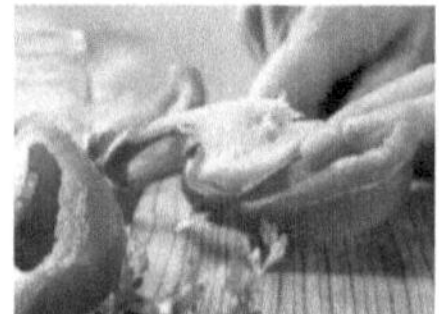

Peppers quarter, core, wash and very finely dice.

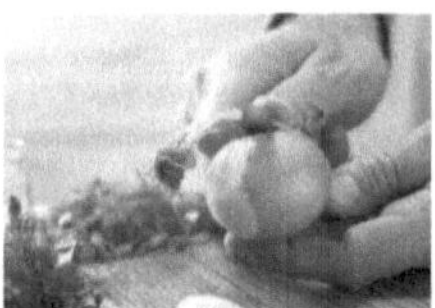

Peel and finely chop the onion and garlic.

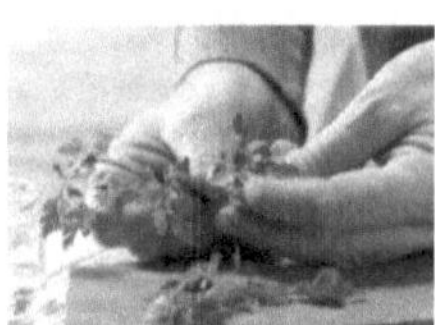

Wash parsley, shake dry, remove leaves and chop finely with a large knife.

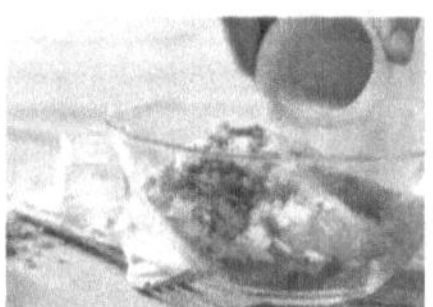

Thoroughly mix the paprika, onions, garlic and parsley with the minced meat, breadcrumbs and quark in a bowl. Season with salt, pepper and cayenne pepper.

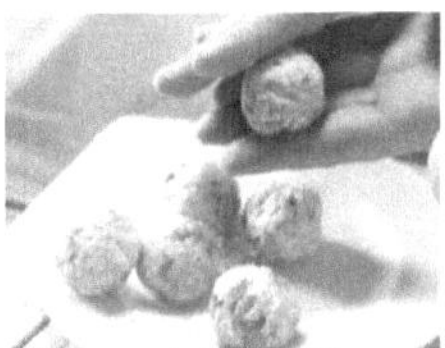

With moistened hands, form 24 small balls from the chopping mass.

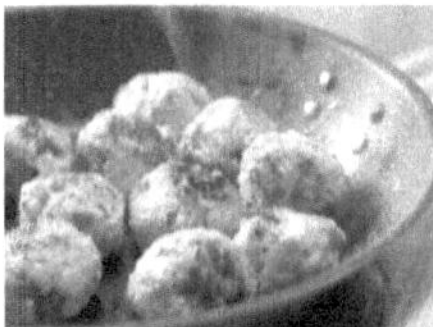

Heat the oil in a large coated pan. Fry the balls until crispy on all sides over medium heat for about 10 minutes, drain on kitchen paper and serve hot or cold.

This recipe is healthy because...

The low-fat, high-protein turkey meat is a good source of vitamins, minerals and trace elements. One portion of the meatballs already covers the daily niacin requirement. The B-vitamin plays a role in nutrient metabolism and contributes to energy production; it also promotes the formation of certain messenger substances in the brain.

Nutritional values

1 Portion contains	(percentage of daily	requirement)
Calories	160 kcal	(8 %)
Protein	27 g	(28 %)
Fat	3 g	(2 %)
Carbohydrates	3 g	(8 %)
added sugar	0 g	(0 %)
Fibres	2 g	(7 %)

Day 2 Lunch

Carrot-ginger soup with orange oil

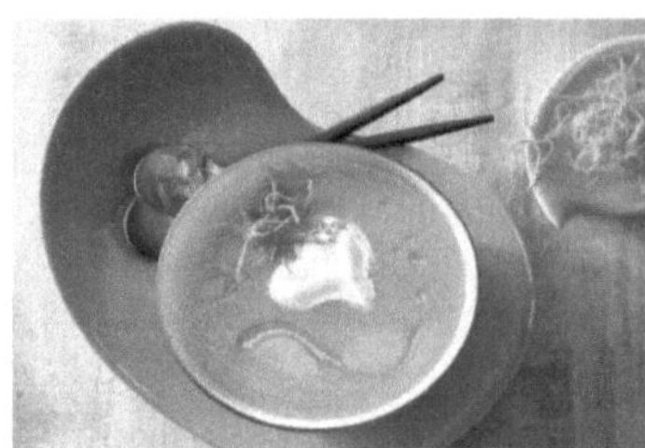

Carrot-ginger soup - A creamy soup with aromatic
spices and a fruity note.

Difficulty: easy
Preparation: 55 Minutes
Calories: 256 kcal

Ingredients for - 2 + portions

1 organic orange
2 tablespoons olive oil (best quality)
300 g carrots (4 carrots)
25 g ginger (1 piece)
2 small shallots
1 tablespoon rapeseed oil
500 ml classic vegetable broth
½ Lemon
Salt
Pepper
50 ml whipped cream

Preparation

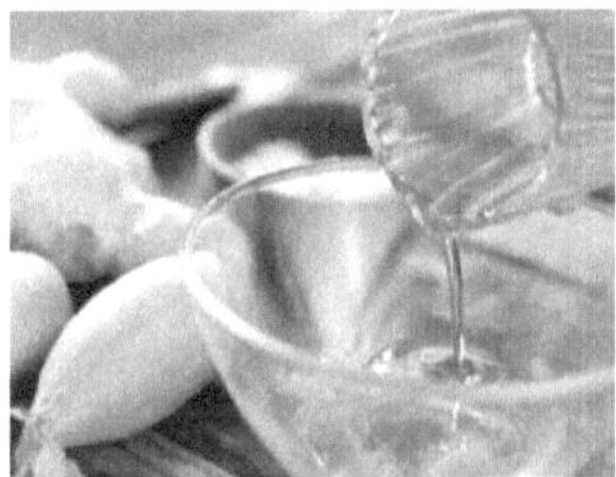

Rinse orange with hot water and rub dry. Finely grate the peel
and mix with the olive oil.

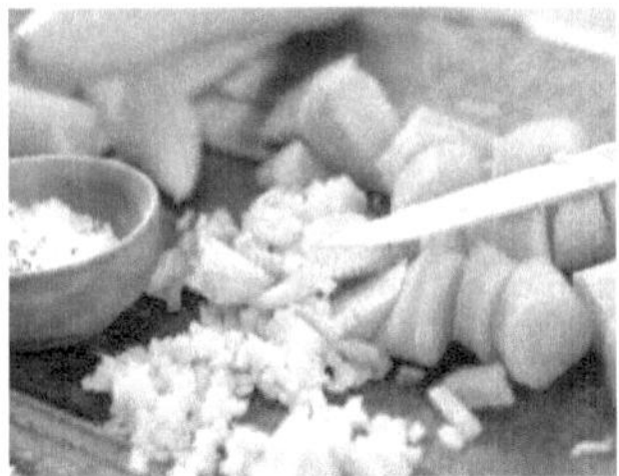

Peel the carrots and cut them into large pieces. Peel and chop the
ginger. Peel the shallots and cut them into fine cubes.

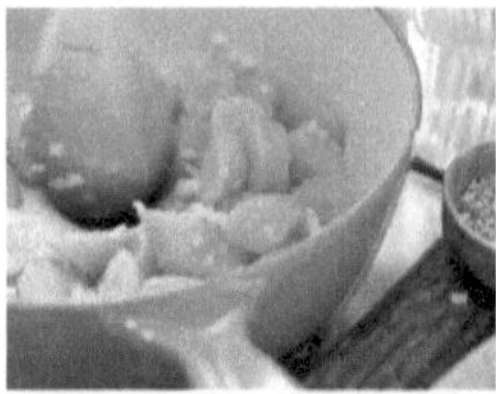

Heat rapeseed oil in a pot. Sauté carrots, ginger and shallots colourlesslyover medium heat.

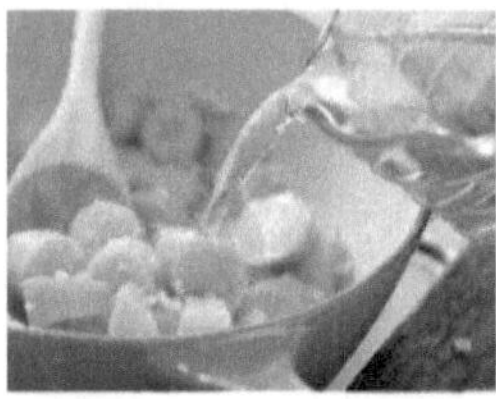

Add the vegetable stock, bring to the boil, cover and cook quietly over medium heat for 25 minutes.

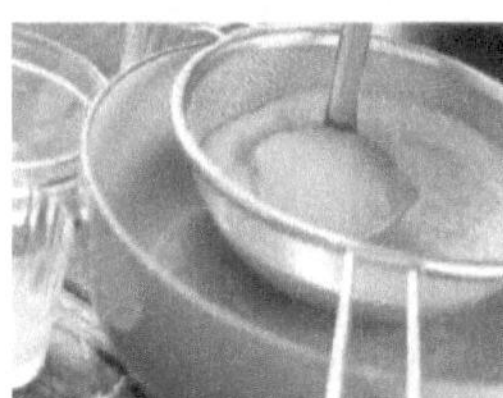

At the end of the cooking time puree the soup very finely with a hand blender and put it through a sieve into a second pot. Squeeze the lemon. Season the carrot-ginger soup with salt, pepper and some lemon juice.

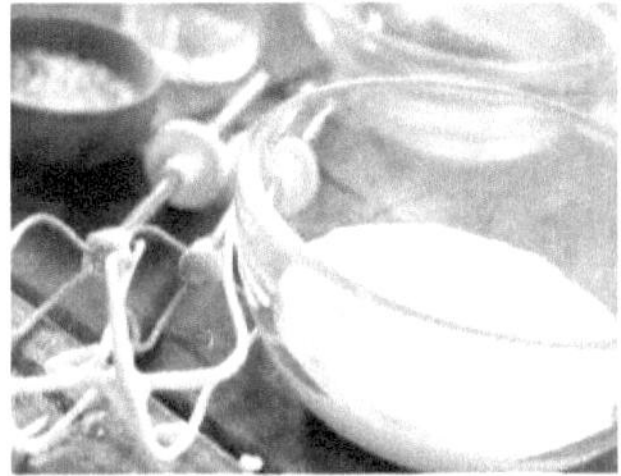

Whip the whipped cream until half stiff.

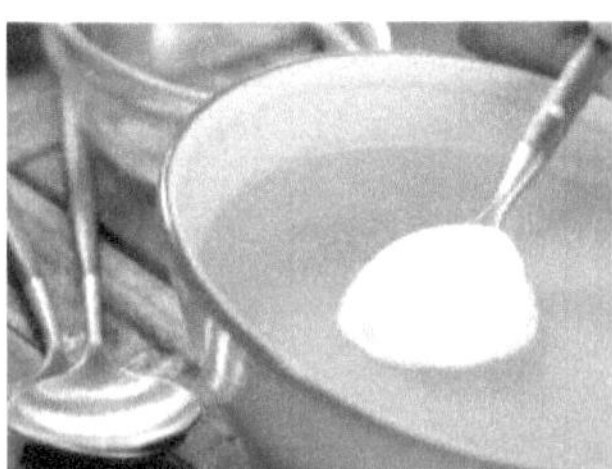

Bring the carrot-ginger soup briefly to the boil again and place in plates. Place 1 tablespoon of cream in the middle of each plate. If you like, form a heart from the cream with a wooden stick.

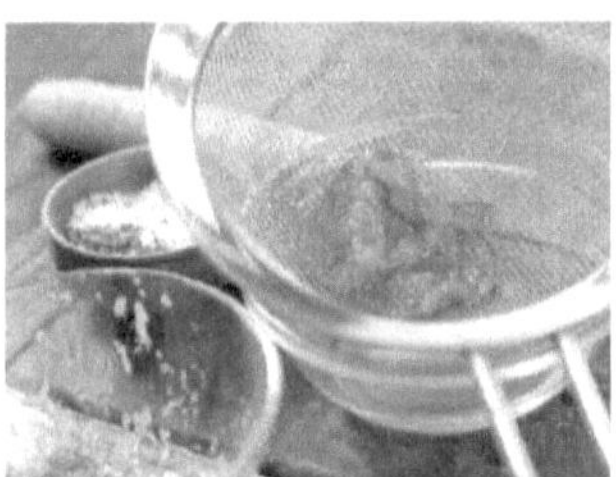

Pass the orange oil through a fine sieve and sprinkle it on the carrot-ginger soup. Crispy fried carrot strips are suitable as garnish.

This recipe is healthy because...

Part of the beta-carotene in the carrots is converted into vitamin A, the rest protects our body cells as an antioxidant. Due to the easily digestible sugar, carrots are also very digestible and are easy on the gastrointestinal tract.

· Nutritional values

1 Portion contains	(percentage of daily	requirement)
Calories	256 kcal	(12 %)
Protein	3 g	(3 %)
Fat	23 g	(20 %)
Carbohydrates	9 g	(6 %)
added sugar	0 g	(0 %)
Fibres	6 g	20 %)

Day 2 Evening meal

Okra curry with fresh coconut

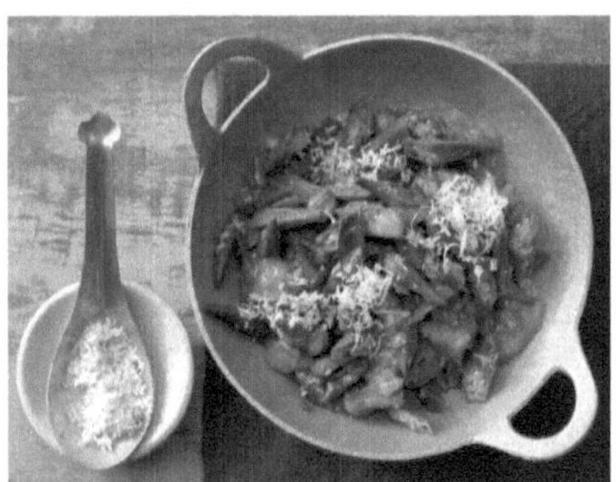

Okra curry with fresh coconut (108 calories per serving) is served in the evening. It is low in carbohydrates and fat. In return, the low-carb dinner scores with a lot of fibre, which ensures good intestinal health and long-lasting satiety.

<u>Difficulty</u>:   easy
<u>Preparation</u>:   20 minutes
<u>Calories</u>:   108 kcal

Ingredients for - 4 + portions

3 shallots
1 piece of fresh coconut (for 50 g pulp)
1 red chilli pepper
500 g okra pods
½ small lime
1 tablespoon rapeseed oil
1 tablespoon light mustard seeds
1 teaspoon curcuma
1 tablespoon cumin seed
10 dried curry leaves
50 ml coconut water
Salt
Pepper

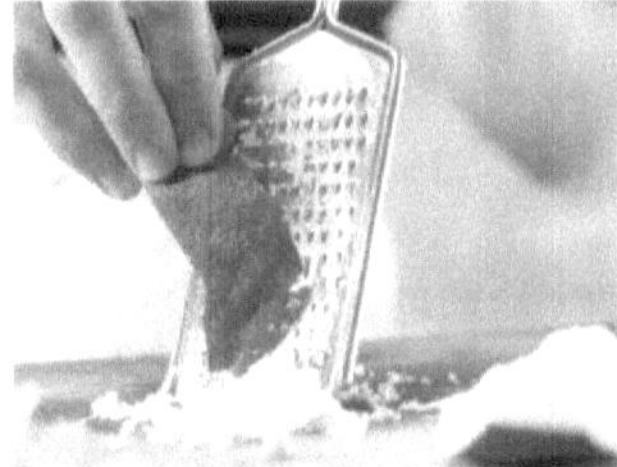

Peel and finely dice the shallots. Peel coconut flesh with a knife or peeler and grate finely.

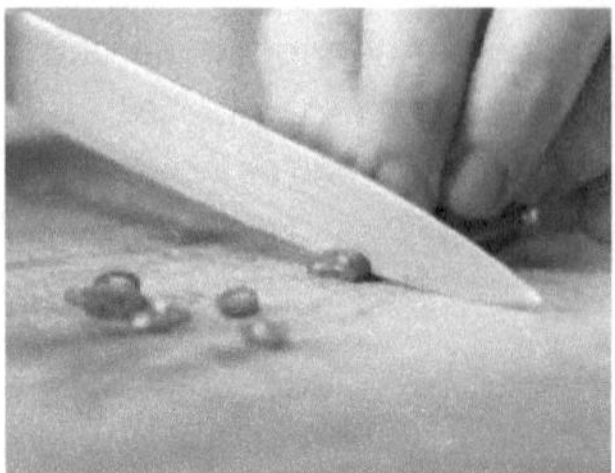

Clean and wash the chili pepper and cut it diagonally into thin slices

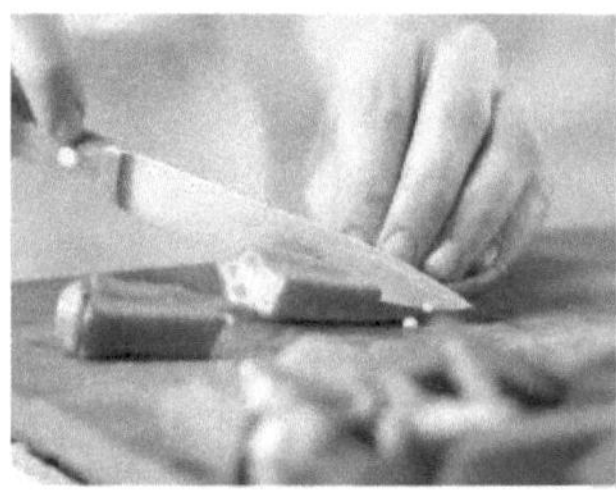

Clean, wash and dry okras and cut them diagonally into 2 cm wide pieces. Squeeze half of the lime.

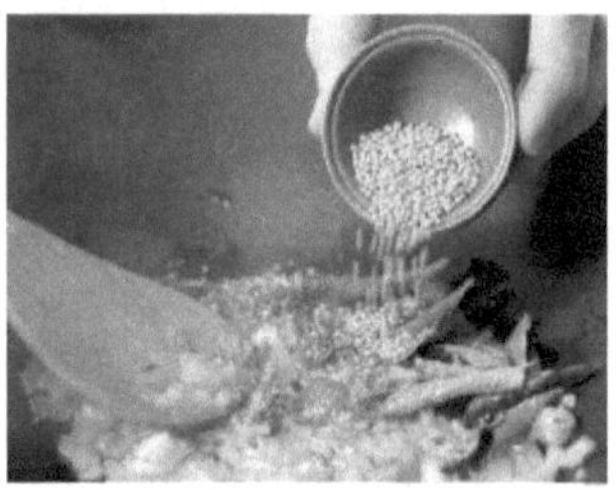

Heat oil in a wok. Sauté the shallots over medium heat until translucent. Add mustard seeds, turmeric, cumin, chili and curry leaves. Stir-fry over a high heat for 2 to 3 minutes.

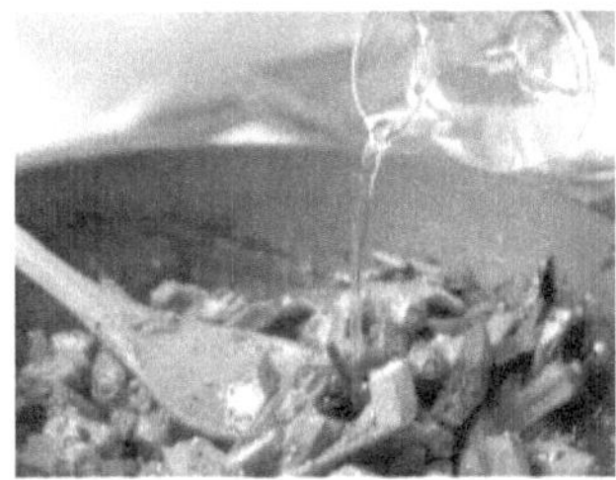

Add the okras and stir-fry for 3 to 4 minutes. Stir in coconut water
And   remove   from   heat.

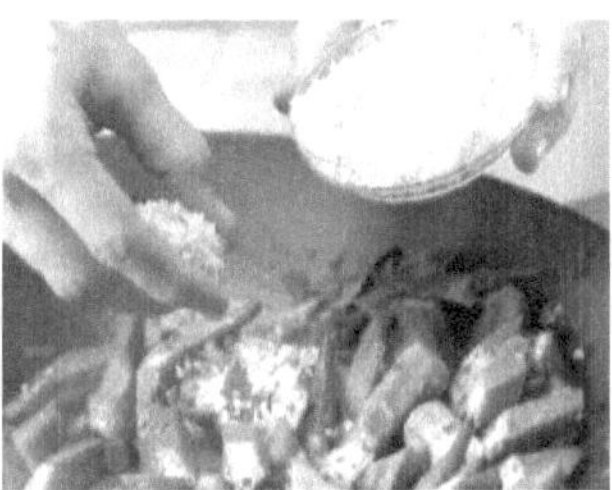

Mix in grated coconut and 1 to 2 tablespoons of lime juice. Salt,
pepper and serve.

This recipe is healthy because...

Every child in Africa, Asia and the Middle East knows them; in our
country okras are still exotic. The mallow plants, which taste a bit like
beans, provide welcome fibre and do not burden the sensationally
low calorie and fat balance in any way.

Nutritional values

1 Portion contains	(percentage of daily	requirement)
Calories	108 kcal	(5 %)
Protein	4 g	(4 %)
Fat	8 g	(3 %)
Carbohydrates	5 g	(6 %)
added sugar	0 g	(0 %)
Fibres	7,5 g	(25 %)

Day 3: Breakfast

Artichoke tortilla with tomatoes and feta cheese

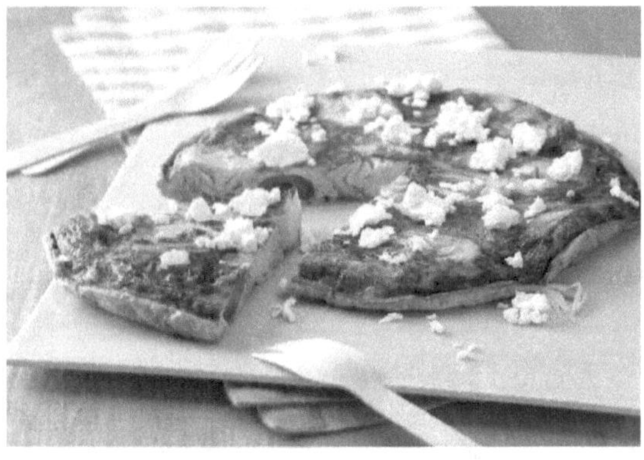

With this delicious pan dish is started in the low-carb Wednesday:
Artichoke tortilla with tomatoes and sheep cheese (246 calories per
serving). Artichokes score points with plenty of fibre to boost
digestion. The eggs provide animal protein, biotin and bone-
strengthening vitamin D. This tortilla tastes hot and cold!

<u>Difficulty</u>:   easy
<u>Preparation</u>:   20 minutes
<u>Calories</u>:   246 kcal

Ingredients for - 2+ portions

220 g artichoke heart (canned; drained weight)
1 onion
1 garlic clove
100 g cherry tomatoes
3 eggs
6 tablespoons of milk (1,5 % fat)
Salt
Pepper
½ TL Tomato paste
1 tsp olive oil
50 g mild sheep's cheese (9 % fat)

Preparation

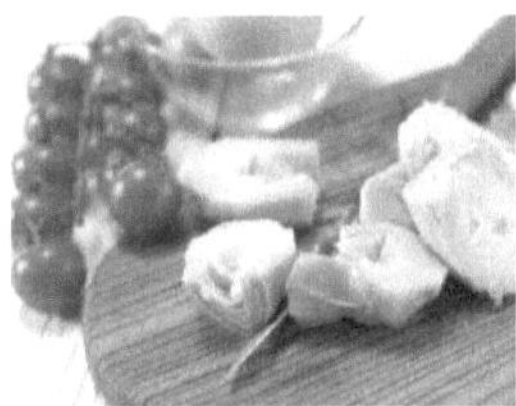

Put artichoke hearts in a sieve, drain well and cut in half.

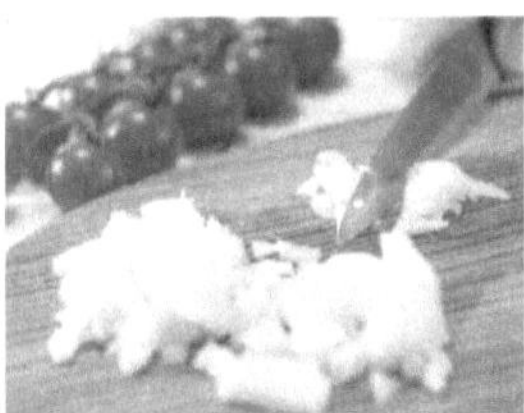

Peel onion and garlic and cut into fine cubes.

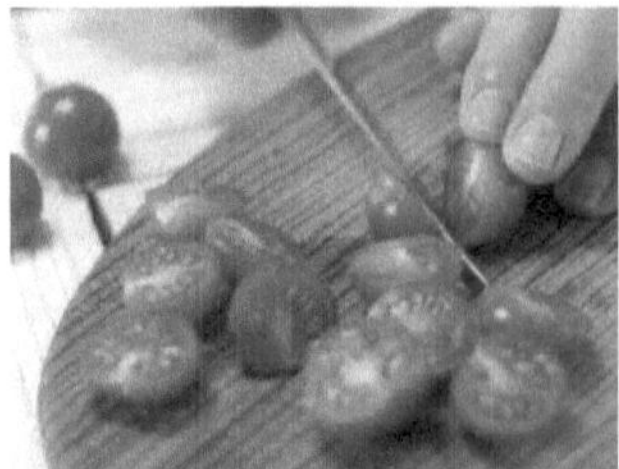

Wash and halve the tomatoe

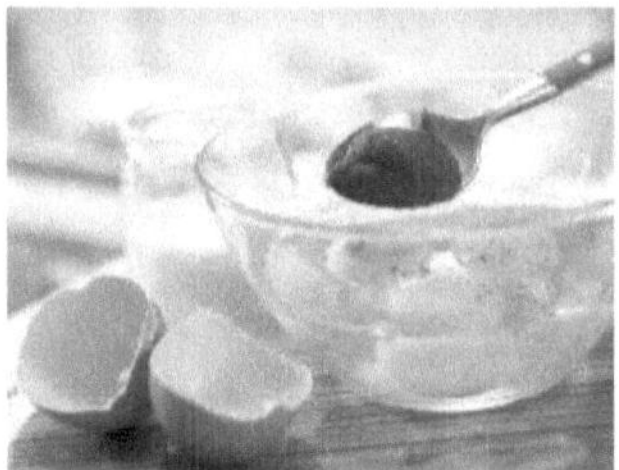

Whisk eggs, milk, salt, pepper and tomato paste

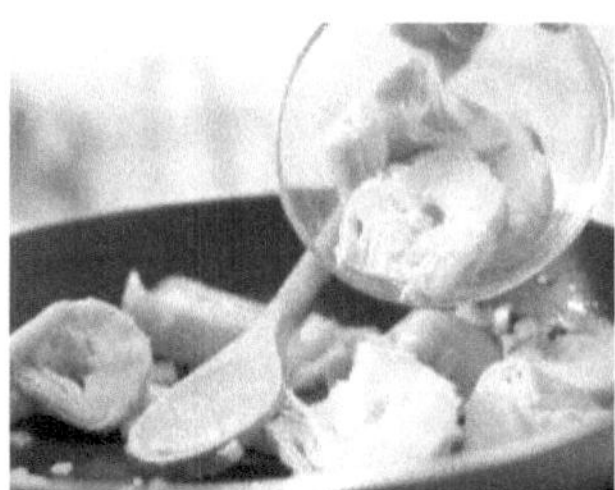

Heat the oil in a coated pan. Fry the onion and garlic over medium heat. Add the artichokes and fry lightly.

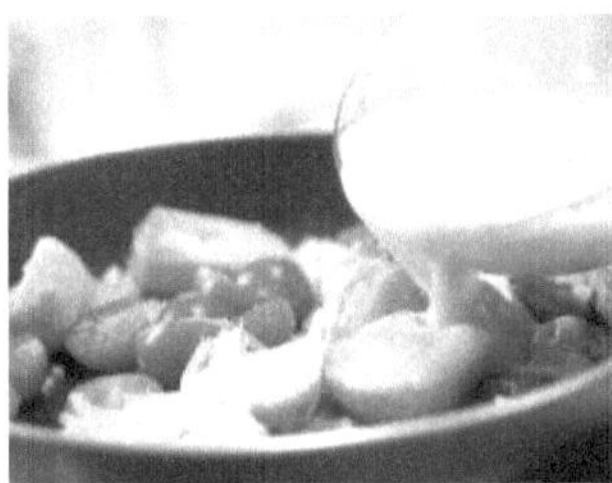

Reduce temperature. Add tomatoes and whisked egg over. Cover and let stand for 6-8 minutes at low heat.

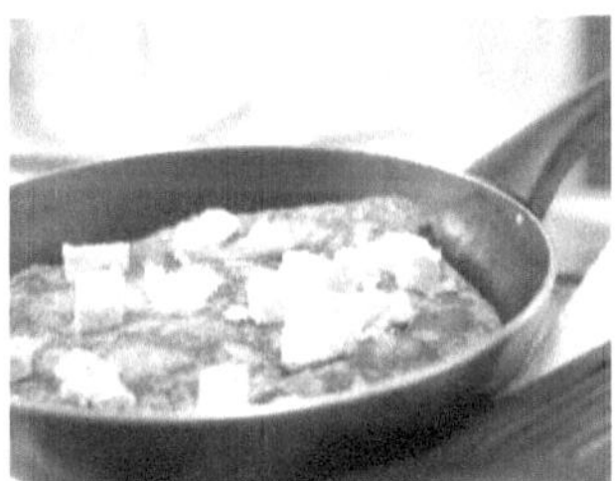

In the meantime cut the cheese into small cubes. Carefully turn the tortilla with a spatula, sprinkle diced sheep's cheese over it and let it melt for a short time. Divide tortilla into pieces. Serve as you like, for example with dark farmhouse bread.

This recipe is healthy because...

Artichokes are the stars among the light ingredients: they are rich in fibre, their vital substances lower blood fat levels and stimulate digestion. The eggs contribute high-quality protein, biotin and bone-strengthening vitamin D - and they cover the daily requirement of vitamin B12.

Nutritional values

1 Portion contains	(percentage of daily	requirement)
Calories	246 kcal	(12 %)
Protein	21 g	(21 %)
Fat	14 g	(12 %)
Carbohydrates	8 g	(9 %)
added sugar	0 g	(0 %)
Fibres	12,5 g	(42 %)

Day 3 Snack
Tofu-peppers-skewers

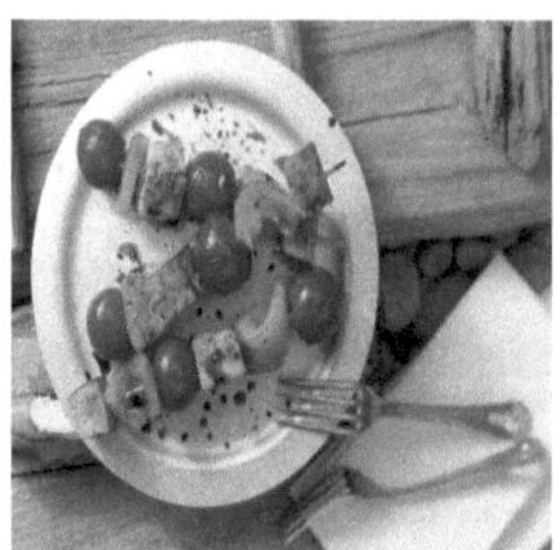

<u>Difficulty:</u>   easy
<u>Preparation:</u> 15 Minutes
<u>Calories:</u>   115 kcal

Ingredients für - 4 + Portions
200 g tofu
1 yellow pepper
100 g cherry tomatoes (8 cherry tomatoes)
Pepper
2 tsp sesame oil

Preparation

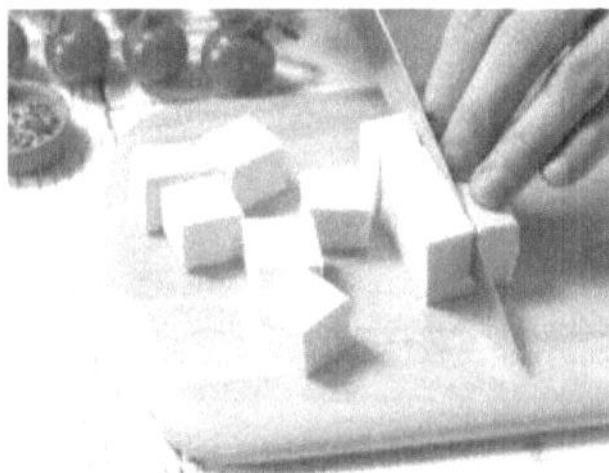

Drain the tofu and cut into cubes of about 2 cm.

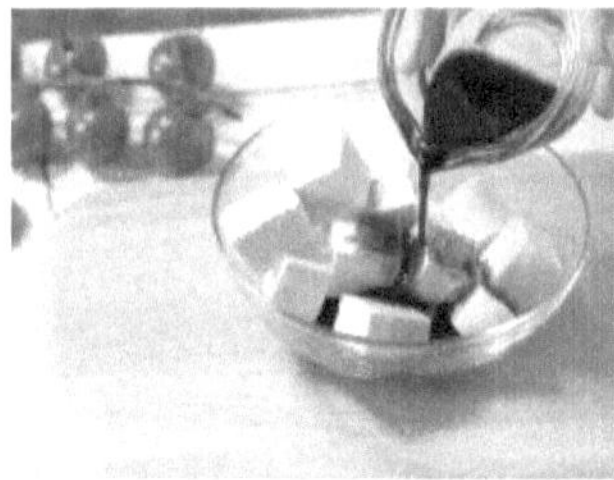

Place the diced tofu in a bowl, mix in the teriyaki sauce and leave
to stand (marinate) for 30 minutes, turning frequently.

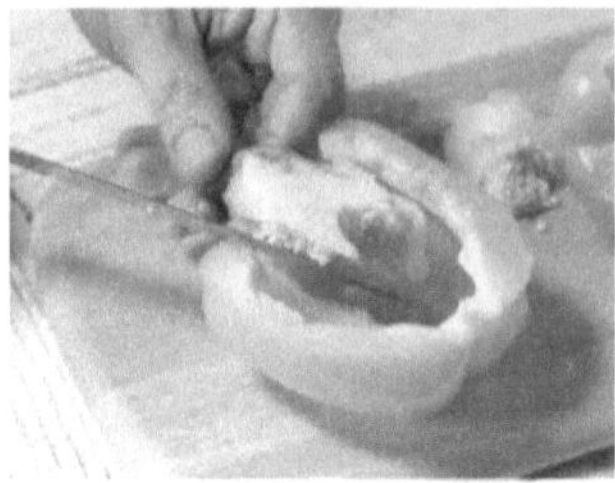

In the meantime, halve the pepper, remove the seeds, wash and cut into even pieces.

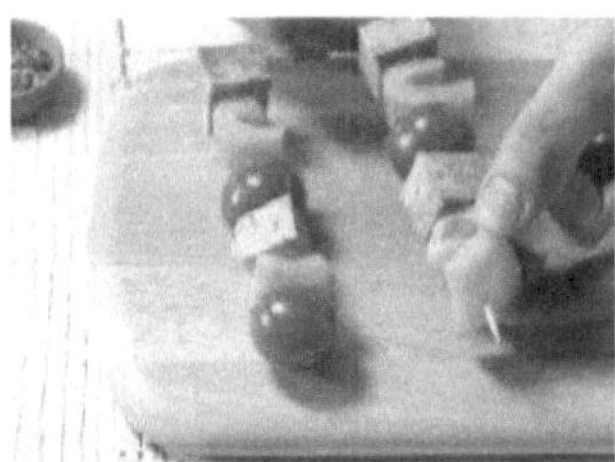

Clean and wash the tomatoes and let them drain in a sieve.

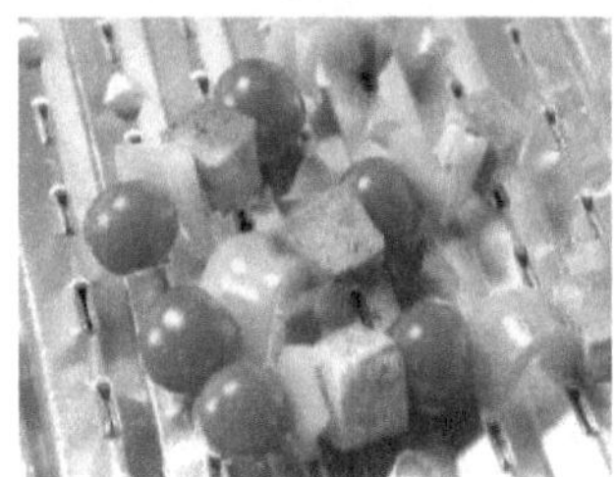

Place on an aluminium grill tray and cook on the hot grill for 6 to 8 minutes, turning occasionally. Pepper the skewers, drizzle with sesame oil and serve.

This recipe is healthy because...

The protein-rich mix of tofu and vegetables has a variety of vitamins and minerals, including iron, a trace element that is often neglected in meat-free diets. Here, however, each portion (= 2 skewers) contains one third of the daily requirement of the mineral which is important for blood formation.

Nutritional values

1 skewer contains	(percentage of daily	requirement)
Calories	115 kcal	(5 %)
Protein	10 g	(10 %)
Fat	6 g	(5 %)
Carbohydrates	3 g	(2 %)
added sugar	0 g	(0 %)
Fibres	3 g	(10 %)

Day 3 Lunch

Fine leaf salad with Bündner meat

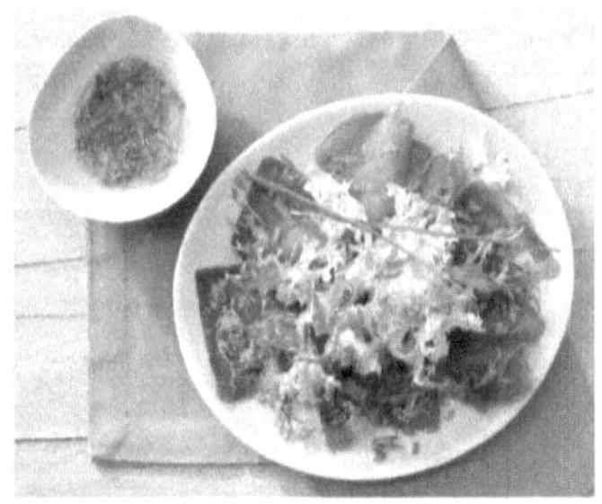

A real delicacy waits in the evening to finally to be eaten: fine leaf salad with Bündner meat (96 calories per serving). Bündner meat is particularly low-fat and contains iron and about 40 percent protein. Nice side effect: This low-carb dinner cranks additionally the fat burning over night.

Difficulty: quite easy
Prepartion: 20 Minutes
Calories: 96 kcal

Ingredients für - 4 + portions

120 g small frisée salad (1 small frisée salad)
250 g lollo bionda (1 lollo bionda)
2 tablespoons cider vinegar
2 tsp. sweet mustard
2 tablespoons Mediterranean vegetable stock
3 tablespoons rapeseed oil
Salt
Pepper
1 bunch of chives
60 g Bündner meat (in wafer-thin slices)

Preparation

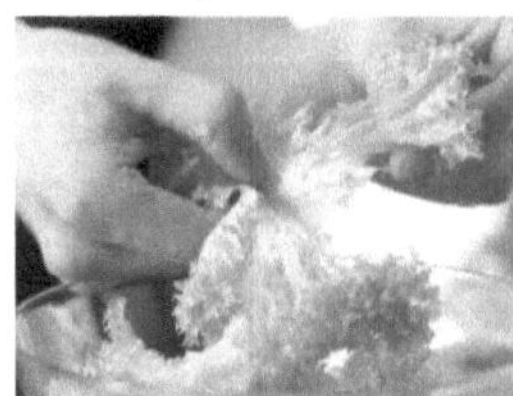

Clean, wash, spin-dry and cut the frisée and lollo bionda into bite-sized pieces. Put them in a large bowl.

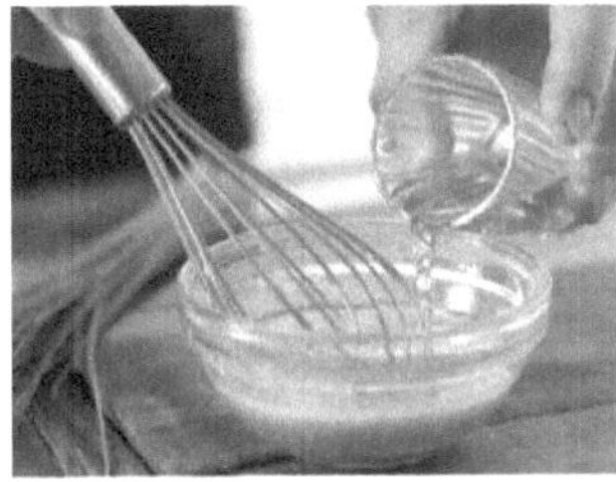

For the dressing, whisk vinegar, mustard, vegetable stock and rapeseed oil in a small bowl with a whisk. Season with salt and pepper.

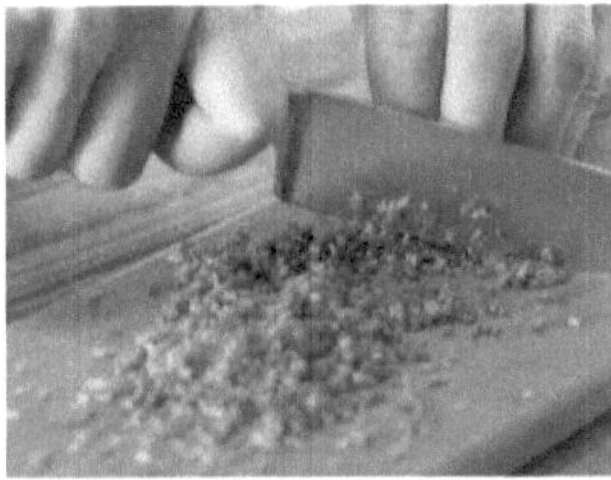

Wash the chives, shake dry, cut into small rolls and add to the dressing. Pour dressing over the salad and mix well

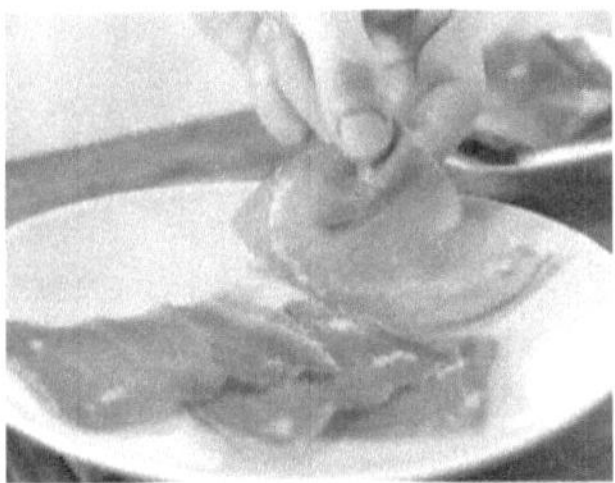

Arrange the Bündner meat in a circle like a carpaccio on flat plates.

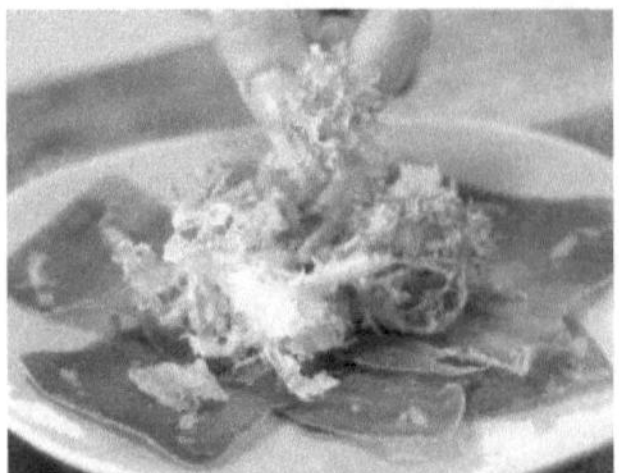

Spread the salad over the meat slices and serve.

This recipe is healthy because...

This pleases figure-conscious connoisseurs: Bündner meat is rightly considered a delicacy on the one hand, but has less than 5 percent fat on the other - and plenty of B vitamins, iron and 40 percent protein. And because it is air-dried, there is hardly any salt in it.

Nutritional values

1 Portion contains	(percentage of daily	requirement)
Calories	96 kcal	(5 %)
Protein	4 g	(4 %)
Fat	8 g	(7 %)
Carbohydrates	1 g	(2 %)
added sugar	0 g	(0 %)
Fibres	1 g	(3 %)

Day 3 Evening meal

Grilled salmon on salad with mustard-honey dressing

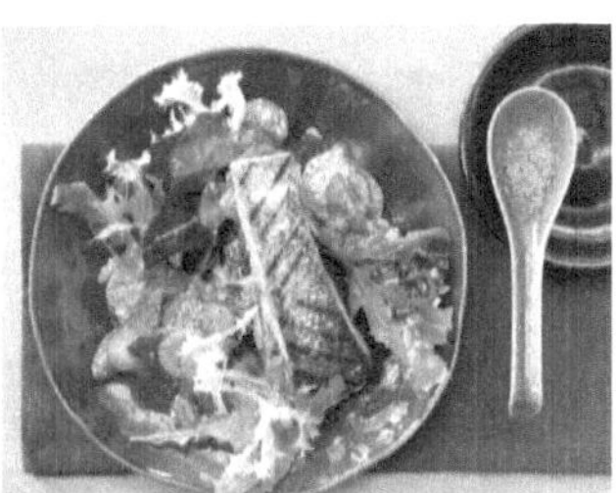

Grilled salmon on salad (318 calories per serving) is served for lunch.
In just 20 minutes, the quick dish is on the table and ready to be
enjoyed. The salmon scores with high-quality protein and
unsaturated fatty acids, which are good for the heart and blood
vessels - and is also a delicious low-carb delicious treat.

Difficulty: easy
Preparation: 10 Minutes
Calories: 318 kcal

Ingredients für - 2 + portions

100 g mixed leaf salad (e.g. frisée, oak leaf, radicchio)
100 g cherry tomatoes
4 radishes
2 salmon fillets (approx. 150 g each, with skin)
Salt
Pepper
2 tablespoons red wine vinegar
1 teaspoon grainy mustard
1 tsp honey
2 tablespoons of olive oil

Preparation

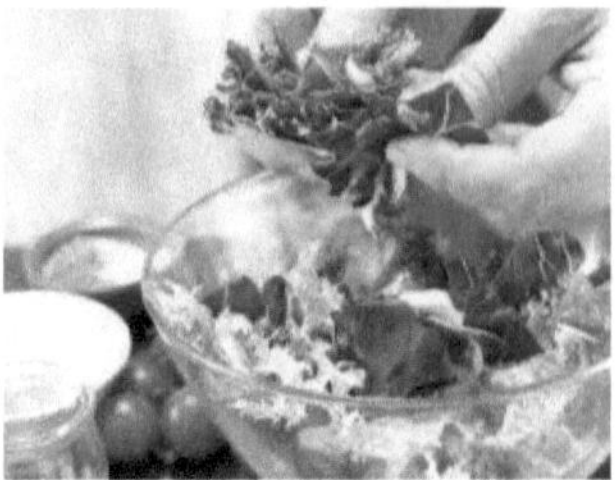

Clean, wash, spin-dry and pluck the salads into bite-sized pieces.

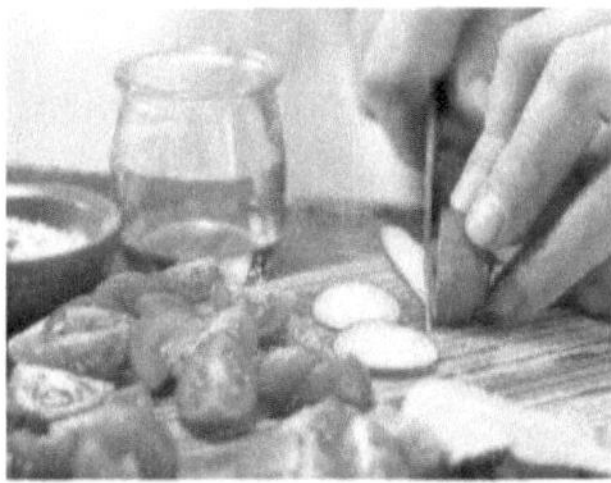

Wash and quarter the cherry tomatoes. Clean and wash the radishes and cut them into thin slices.

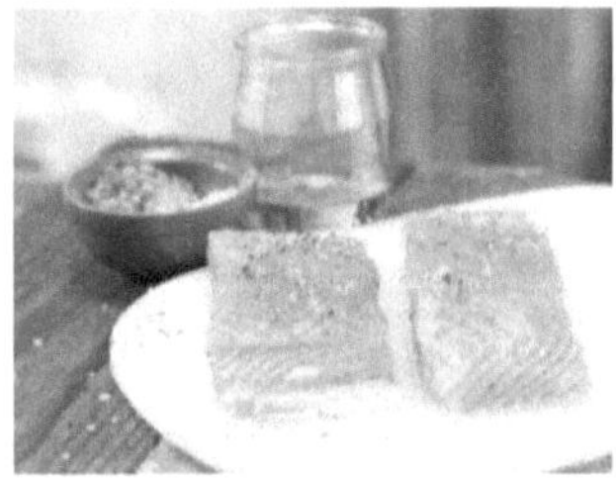

Wash the salmon fillets, dab dry with kitchen paper and season with salt and pepper.

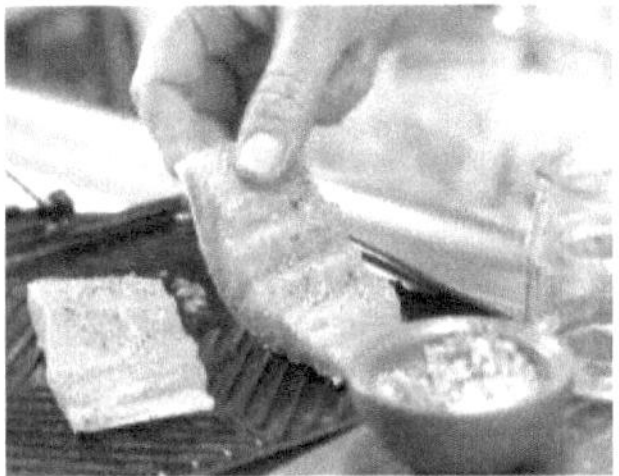

Heat a grill pan and fry the salmon fillets in it on the skin side for
5 to 6 minutes at medium heat.

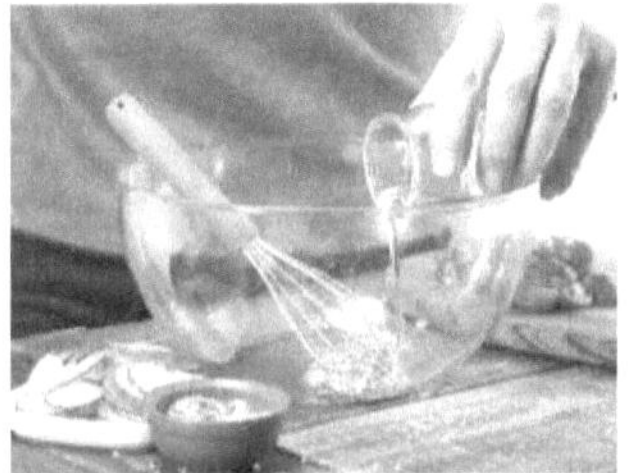

In the meantime, whisk the vinegar in a large bowl with 2 tablespoons
of water, mustard, honey and oil to make a dressing. Season with
salt and pepper

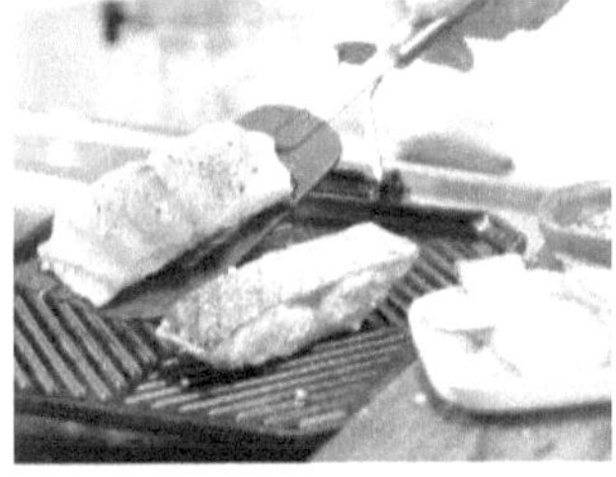

Turn salmon fillets and fry on the meat side for 1 to 2 minutes

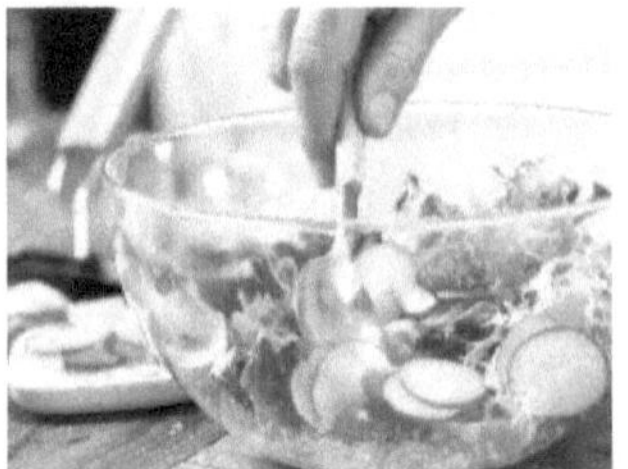

Mix the tomatoes, radishes and lettuce with the dressing and serve with the salmon fillets.

This recipe is healthy because...

Almost everyone loves salmon - and that's a good thing, because the formerly so expensive noble fish provides not only plenty of protein but also unsaturated fatty acids, which are useful for the heart and blood vessels, as well as various vitamins: One portion easily covers the daily requirement of vitamin B6 and B12.

Nutritional values

1 Portion contains	(percentage of daily	requirement)
Calories	318 kcal	(15 %)
Protein	36 g	(37 %)
Fat	14 g	(3 %)
Carbohydrates	5 g	(13 %)
added sugar	0 g	(0 %)
Fibres	1,5 g	(5 %)

Day 4 Breakfast

Pecorino cheese with vegetables and mint

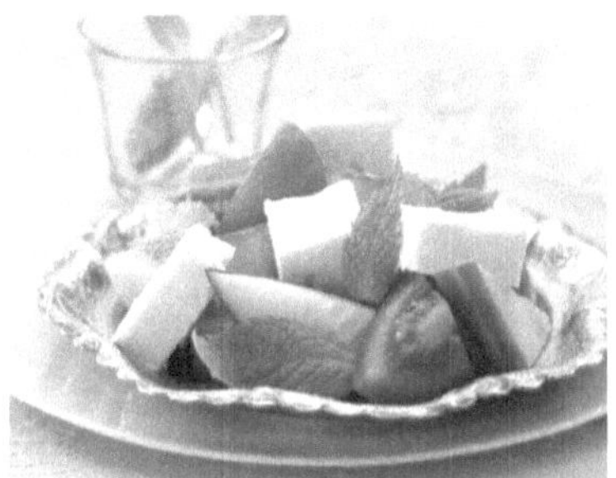

Pecorino cheese with vegetables and mint (80 calories per serving)
is on the breakfast table in no time at all and is the prelude to the
low-carb diet on Thursday. The crunchy vegetables provide valuable
vitamins, minerals and fibre. In addition, the mint adds a fresh flavour
to the dish and makes it even easier to digest.

Difficulty: quiet easy
Preparation: 10 Minutes
Calories: 80 kcal

Ingredients for - 1 + portion

80 g tomatoes (1 tomato)
80 g cucumber (1 piece)
50 g feta cheese (9 % fat)
1 stalk of mint

Preparation

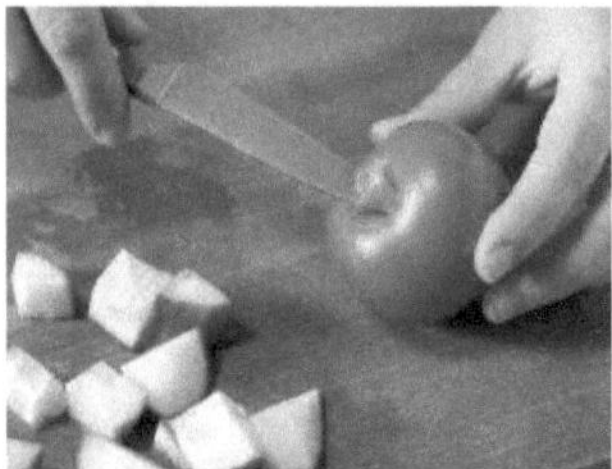

Wash the tomato and cucumber and rub dry. Cut out the stalk of
the tomato in a wedge shape. Cut the tomato and cucumber into
cubes.

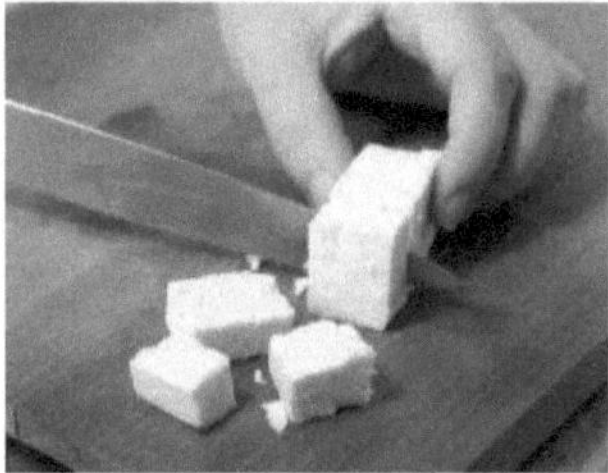

Cut sheep's cheese into cubes as well. Wash the mint, shake dry
and remove the leaves. Arrange vegetables, cheese and mint on
a plate.

This recipe is healthy because...

This is how a low-calorie snack must be: appetizing, crunchy and
naturally rich in nutrients. With only 5 grams of fat and a whole 80
calories of protein, fibre and vitamins, this snack is full!

Nutritional values

1 Portion contains	(percentage of daily	requirement)
Calories	80 kcal	(4 %)
Protein	5 g	(5 %)
Fat	4 g	(2 %)
Carbohydrates	3 g	(7 %)
added sugar	0 g	(0 %)
Fibres	1 g	(3 %)

Day 4 Snack

Baked spinach nests with egg

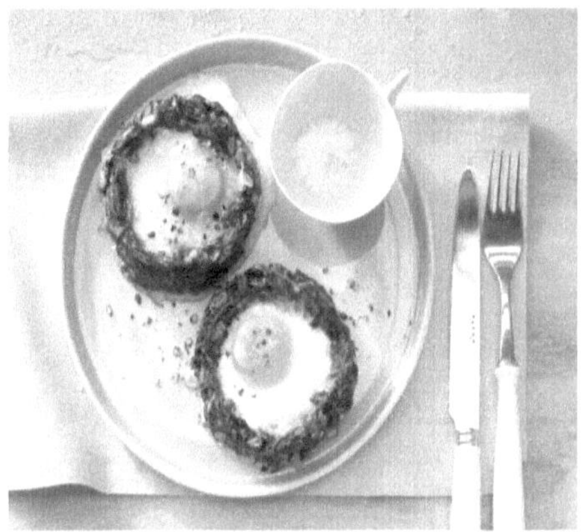

This protein-rich low-carb snack not only looks good, but also
contains vitamin A and lots of iron: the baked spinach nests (178
calories per serving). If you use deep-frozen spinach, you should
squeeze it out thoroughly after defrosting so that the excess
condensation escapes and the nests are better kept.

Difficulty: medium
Preparation: 25 Minutes
Calories: 178 kcal

Ingredients for - 4 + portions

1 garlic clove
1 onion
1 kg fresh leaf spinach
2 tablespoons rapeseed oil
Nutmeg
Salt
Pepper
4 eggs

Preparation

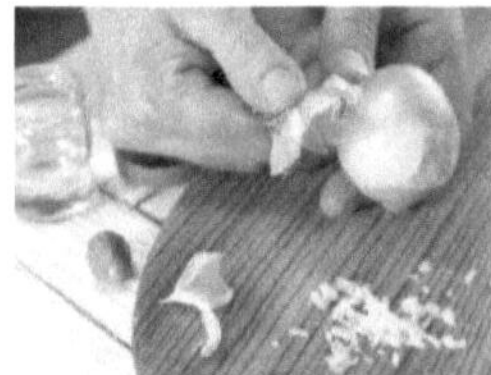

Peel garlic and onion and dice very finely.

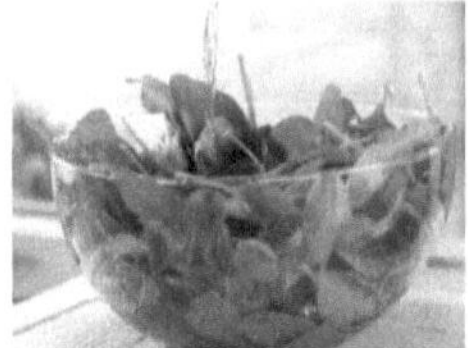

Clean the spinach, wash it thoroughly and let it drip off slightly in a sieve.

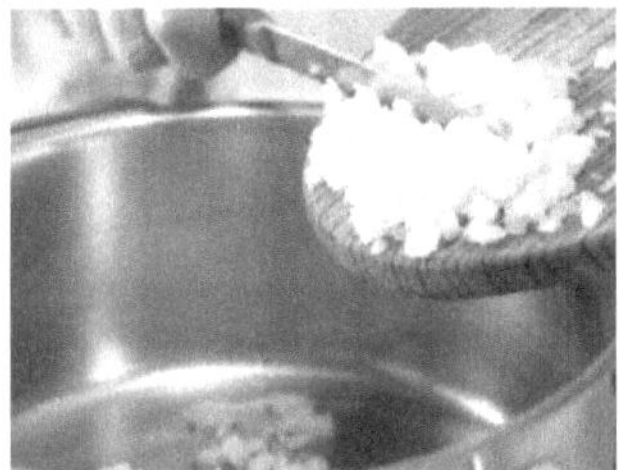

Heat rapeseed oil in a pot, fry onion and garlic over medium heat until transparent.

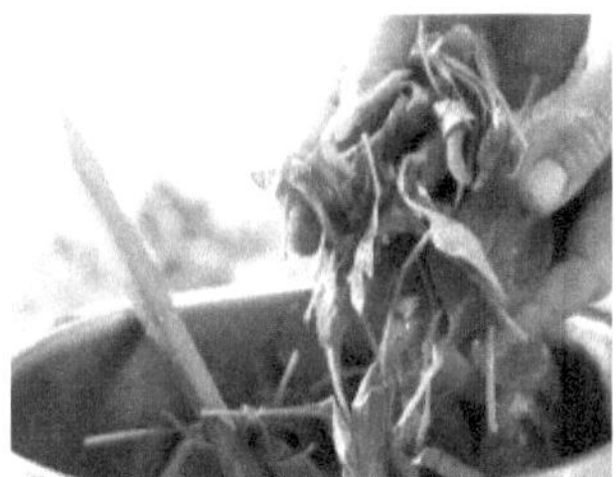

Add the spinach dripping wet and let it collapse while stirring. Rub in a little nutmeg and season with salt and pepper.

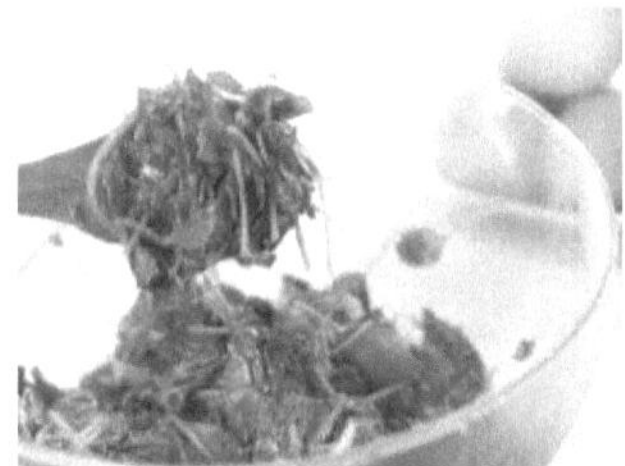

Put the spinach in a bowl and let it cool down a little.

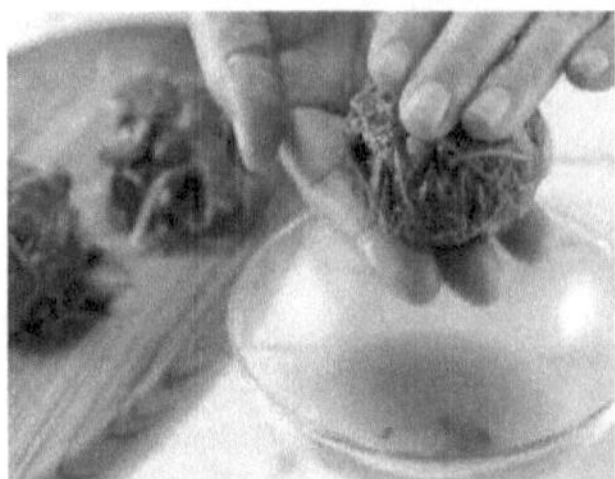

Divide the spinach into 4 portions. Shape into 4 firm balls with your hands, squeezing well over a bowl. Line a baking tray with baking paper.

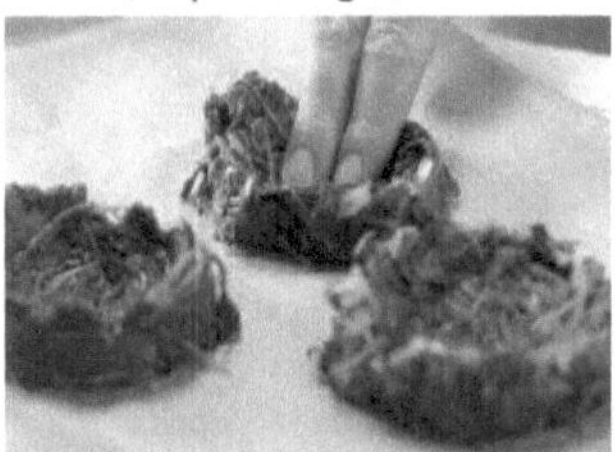

Place the spinach balls on the baking tray. First press flat, then form a depression in the middle of each ball.

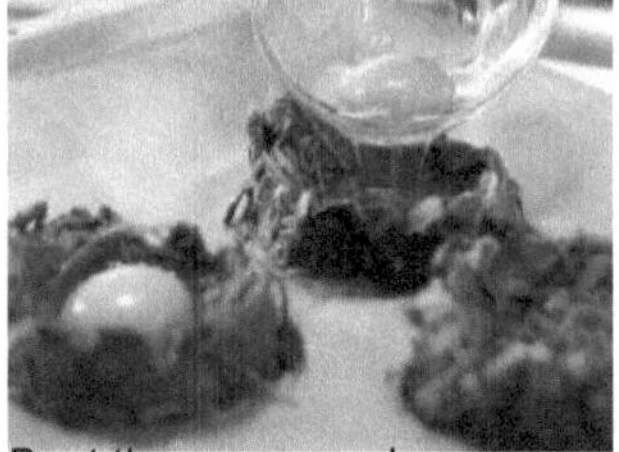

Beat the eggs one by one over a small bowl and slide one into each well.

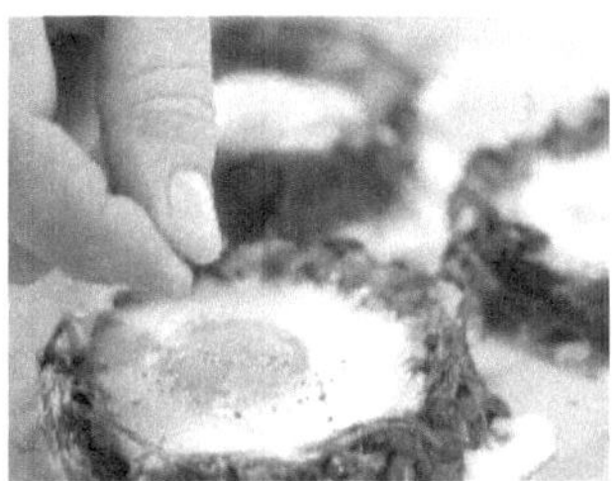

Bake the spinach nests in a preheated oven at 200 °C (fan oven 180 °C, gas mark 3) on the 2nd rack from below for 15 to 20 minutes. Season with salt and pepper.

This recipe is healthy because...

Anyone who takes hold here does something for perspective and strength: the pretty nests provide two and a half times the daily requirement of vitamin A and more than half of the daily required amount of iron.

Nutritional values

1 Portion contains	(percentage of daily	requirement)
Calories	178 kcal	(8 %)
Protein	13 g	(13 %)
Fat	10 g	(1 %)
Carbohydrates	2 g	(8 %)
added sugar	0 g	(0 %)
Fibres	6 g	(20 %)

Day 4 Lunch
Chicken fricassee with asparagus and mushrooms

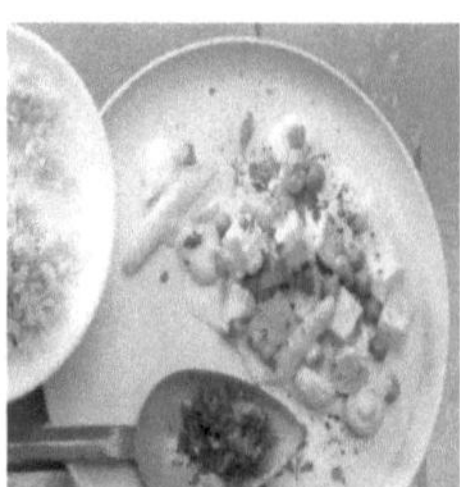

Chicken fricassee (340 calories per serving) is served for lunch with the low-carb nutrition plan. The chicken fricassee contains few calories, but provides high-quality animal protein. In addition, vitamins B12 and B6 stimulate the energy metabolism. This classic meal will keep you full for a long time and you can eat a lot.

Difficulty: easy
Preparation: 50 Minutes
Calories: 340 kcal

Ingredients for - 4 + Portions

900 g double chicken breast on the bone (2 double chicken breasts)
3 onions
1 bunch of soup greens
Salt
1 bay leaf
10 black peppercorns
250 ml soy cream
400 g white asparagus
200 g small mushrooms
100 g peas (frozen)
½ Lemon
Nutmeg
Pepper   Chervil to taste (for garnishing)

Preparation

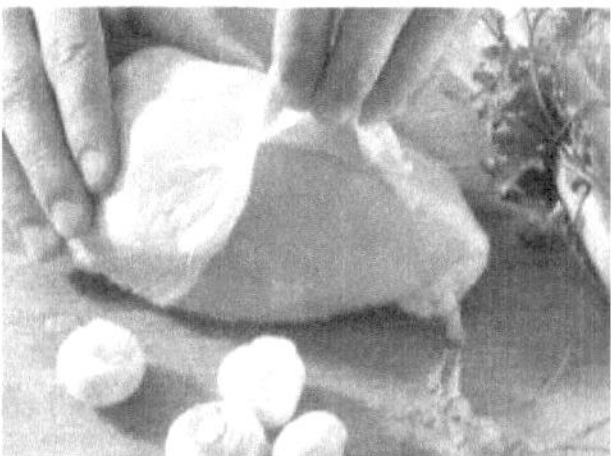

Wash the chicken, dab dry and remove the skin. Bring chicken breasts to the boil in 1.2 l water with very little salt. Skim off any foam with a skimmer.

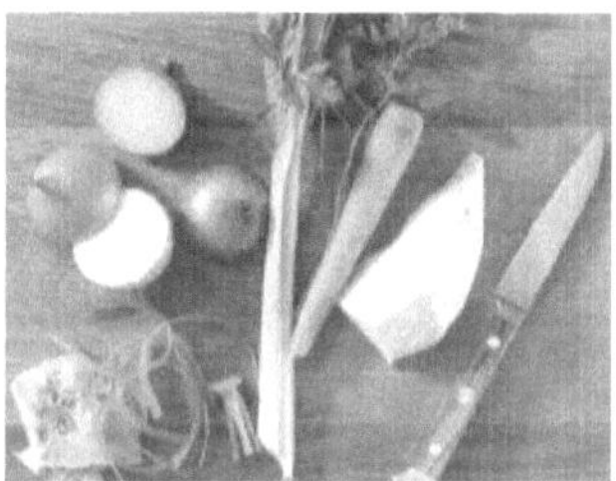

In the meantime, cut the onions in half unpeeled. Clean the soup greens, peel the carrot and celery and chop everything up.

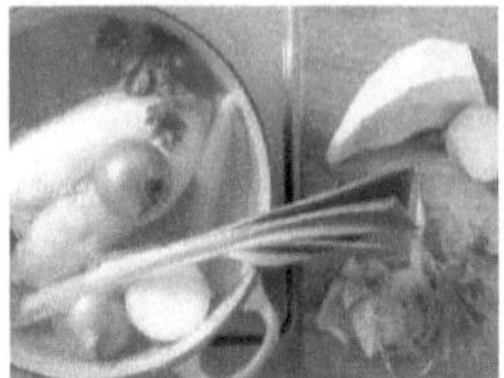

Add onions and soup vegetables together with bay leaf and peppercorns to the chicken and cook over medium heat for 35 minute

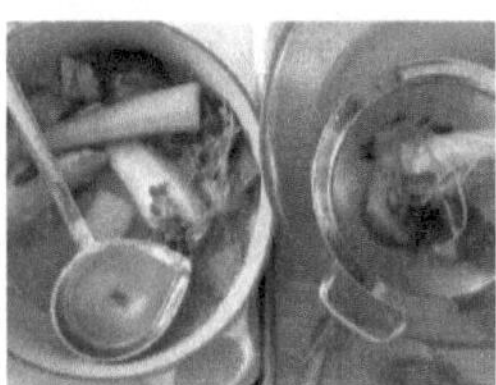

Remove the chicken breast from the pot and set aside.
Pass the stock through a sieve and collect.

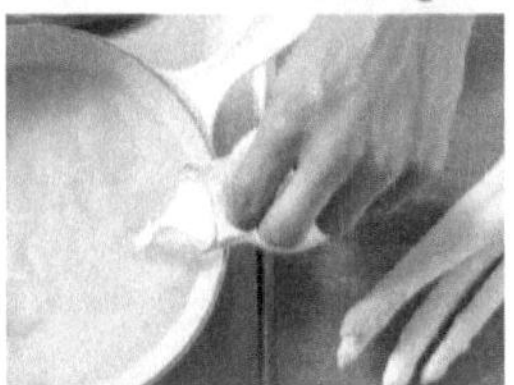

Measure 750 ml stock and bring to the boil with the soy cream. Boil down to 550 ml over a high heat in 15 to 20 minutes

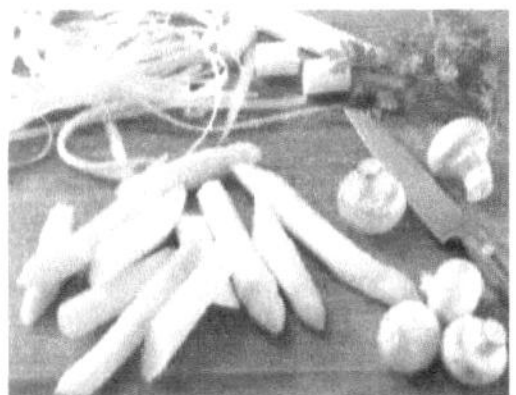

In the meantime, wash and peel the asparagus and cut off the woody ends. Cut the stalks into 4 cm long pieces.

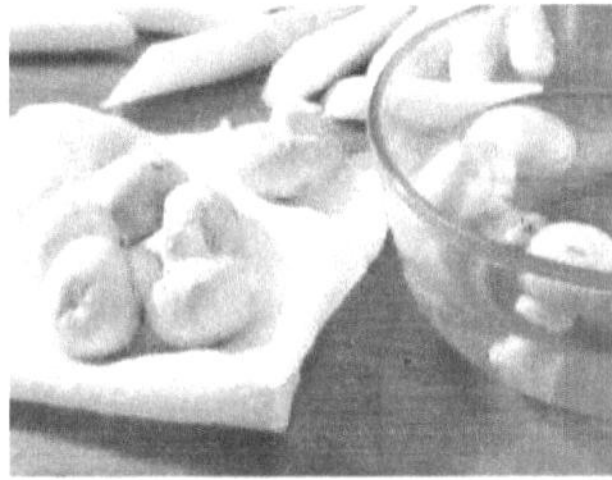

Wash, clean, drain and halve the mushrooms.

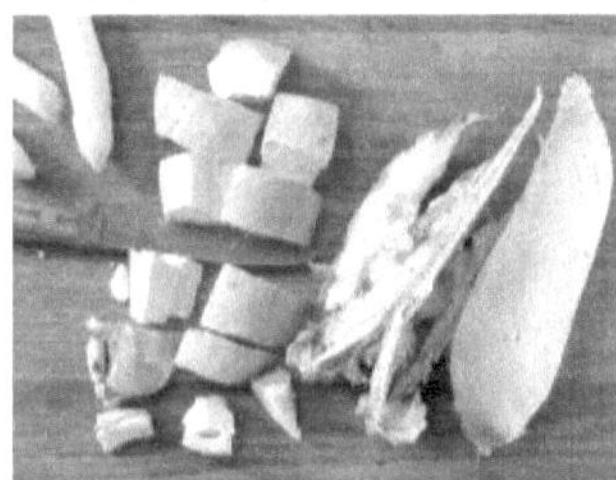

Remove the chicken meat from the bones and cut into 2 cm cubes.

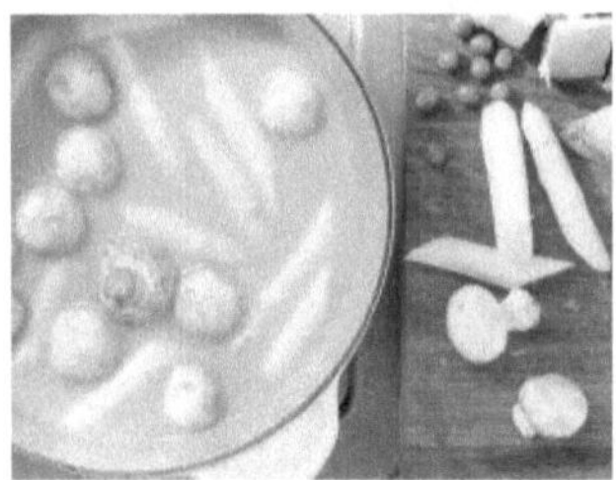

Add the asparagus and mushrooms to the boiled stock in the pot and cook over a medium heat for 10 minutes.

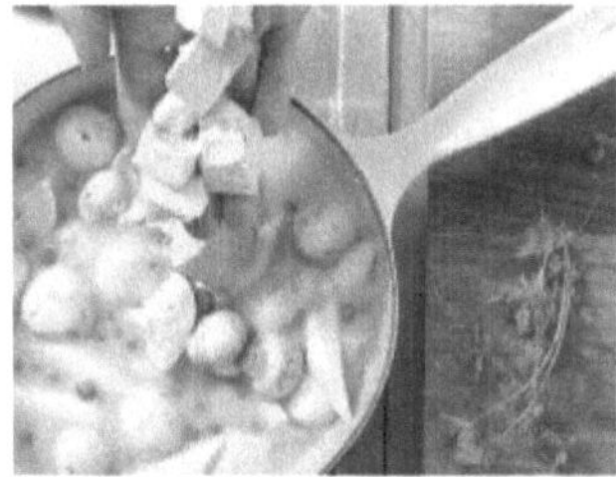

Add peas and meat and cook for another 3 minutes. Squeeze the lemon and grate some nutmeg. Season the chicken fricassee with salt, pepper, nutmeg and lemon juice and garnish with some chervil as desired.

This recipe is healthy because...

Chicken fricassee is low in calories and provides high-quality protein and plenty of B vitamins: Vitamin B6, pantothenic acid and niacin ensure smooth energy metabolism and strong nerves.

Nutritional values

1 Portion contains	(percentage of daily	requirement)
Calories	340 kcal	(16 %)
Protein	48 g	(49 %)
Fat	12 g	(10 %)
Carbohydrates	7 g	(22 %)
added sugar	0 g	(0 %)
Fibres	4,5 g	(15 %)

Day 4 Evening meal

baked parsnips with almonds and rosemary

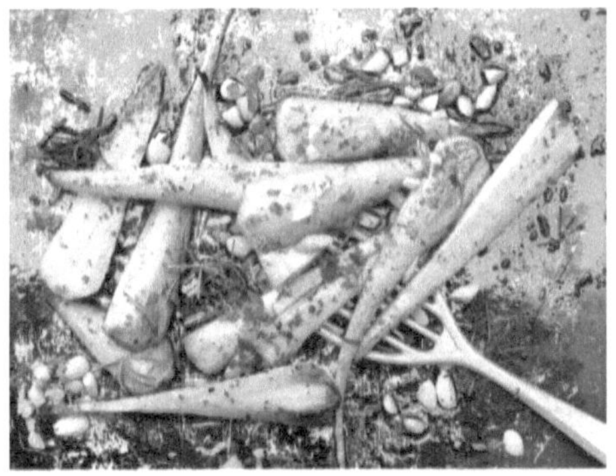

Pre-heat the oven, because on Thursday evening baked parsnips with almonds and rosemary (192 calories per serving) will be served. The well-known root vegetable is being rediscovered by Foodies and is landing on plates more and more often. Parsnips are a good low-carb vegetable because they are dehydrating, low in carbohydrates and contain many B vitamins.

Difficulty: easy
Preparation: 25 Minutes
Calories: 192 kcal

Ingredients for – 4 + portions

650 g Parsnips
1 Branch of rosemary
3 tbsp. olive oil
1tbsp. liquid honey
Salt
Pepper
75 g unpeeled almonds
3 Branch Parsley

Preparation

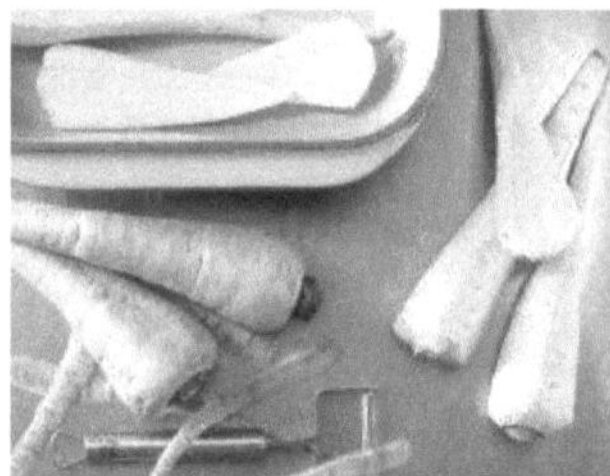

Wash and clean the parsnips and peel them generously with a peeler. Depending on the thickness, cut lengthwise in half or quarters and place in a large bowl.

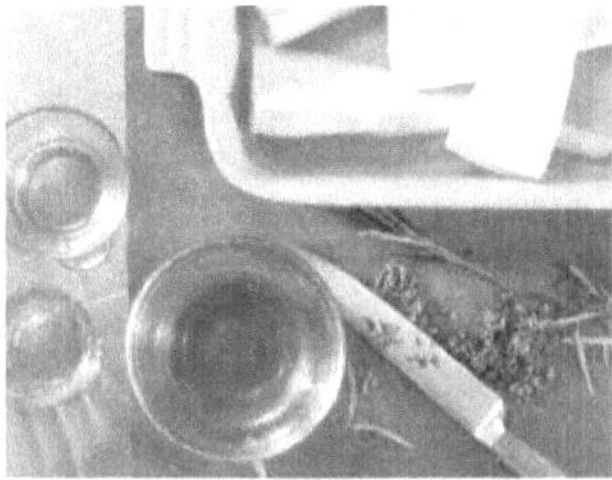

Wash the rosemary, shake dry, remove the needles and chop finely. In a small bowl, mix oil, honey and a little salt and pepper.

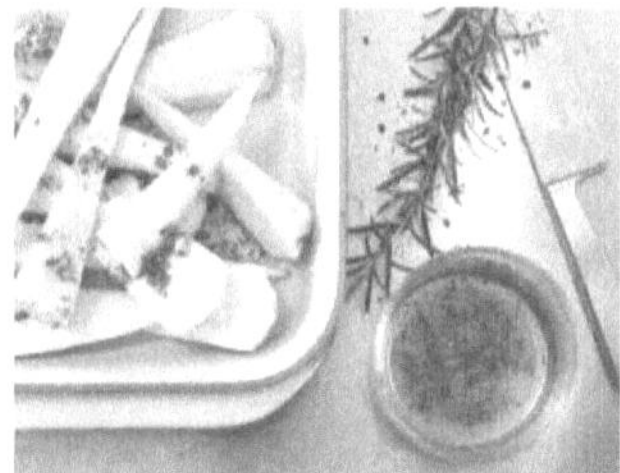

Pour the seasoning oil over the parsnips and mix everything well.

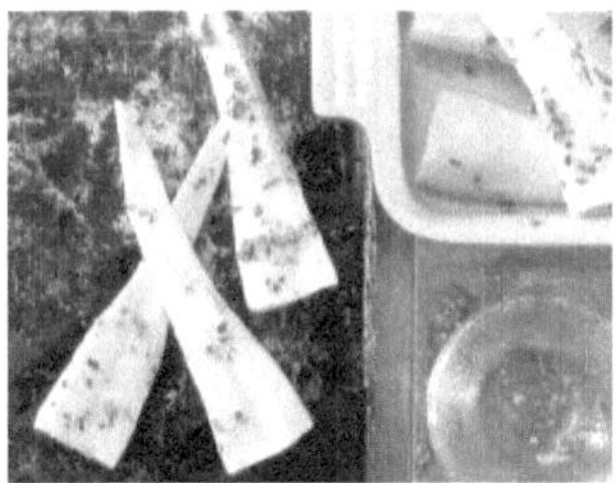

Put the parsnips with the seasoning oil on a baking tray.

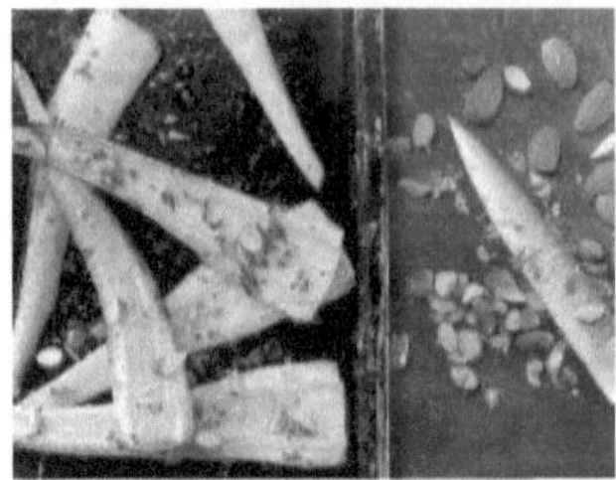

Bake in a preheated oven at 200 °C (fan oven: not recommended, gas: level 3) on the 2nd rack from below for 25 minutes, turning once after 15 minutes. Chop the almonds and sprinkle over the vegetables after 20 minutes.

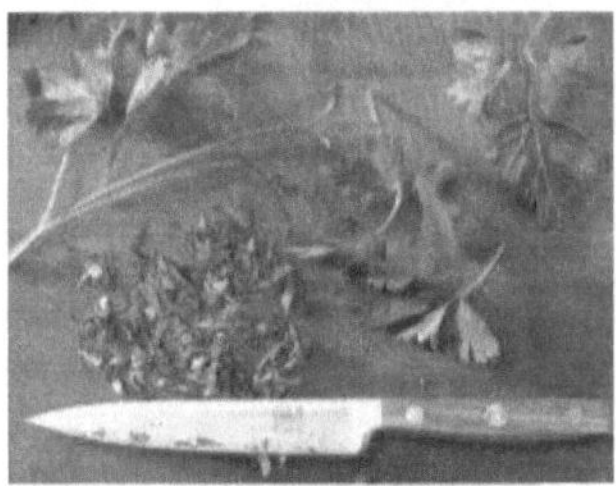

Wash parsley, shake dry, pluck off leaves and chop. Sprinkle over the baked parsnips and serve. Goes well with poultry or short roasted meat.

This recipe is healthy because...

Time to rediscover the somewhat forgotten roots! After all, parsnips offer - in addition to their spicy taste - several vitamins of the B group and, in addition, plenty of potassium with a draining effect.

Nutritional values

1 Portion contains	(percentage of daily	requirement)
Calories	192 kcal	(9 %)
Protein	5 g	(5 %)
Fat	15 g	(13 %)
Carbohydrates	7 g	(17 %)
added sugar	3 g	(12 %)
Fibres	9 g	(30 %)

Day 5 Breakfast
Foam omelette with leaf spinach and sprouts

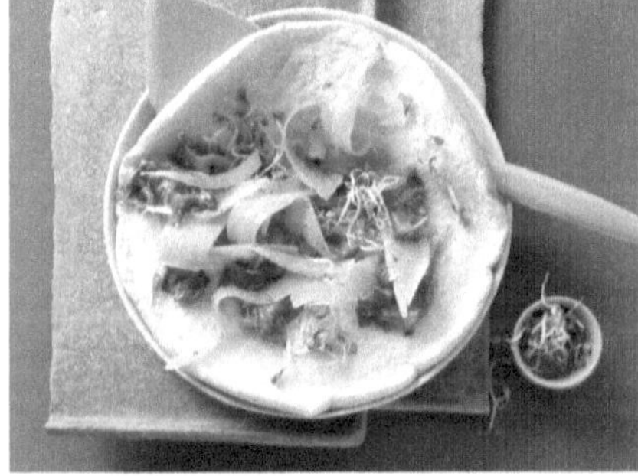

On the low-carb morning meal plan is the delicious foam omelette with leaf spinach and sprouts (310 calories per serving). This is particularly airy and light and a good source of protein. This dish also contains minerals and vitamins: Vitamin E in particular is contained in this omelette, which protects the cells from free radicals.

<u>Difficulty:</u>   easy
<u>Preparation:</u> 15 Minutes
<u>Calories:</u>   210 kcal

Ingredients for – 2 + portions

250 g fennel bulb (1 fennel bulb)
1 ½ Tbsp. germ oil
Salt
150 g leaf spinach (deep-frozen)
4 eggs
100 g carrots (1 carrot)
Pepper
40 g sprouts (e.g. radish sprouts)

Preparation

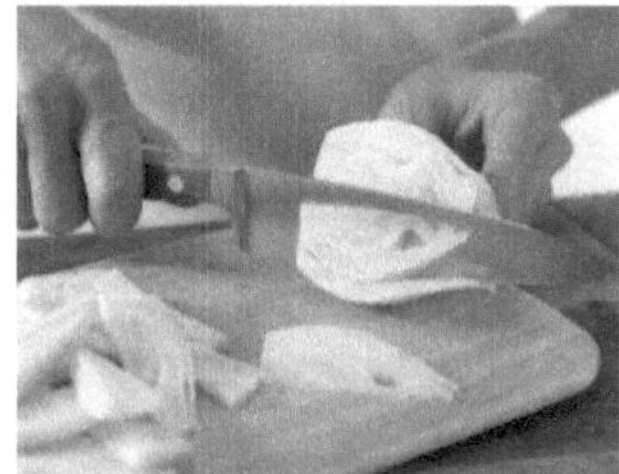

Fennel wash, clean, halve and cut into narrow slices.

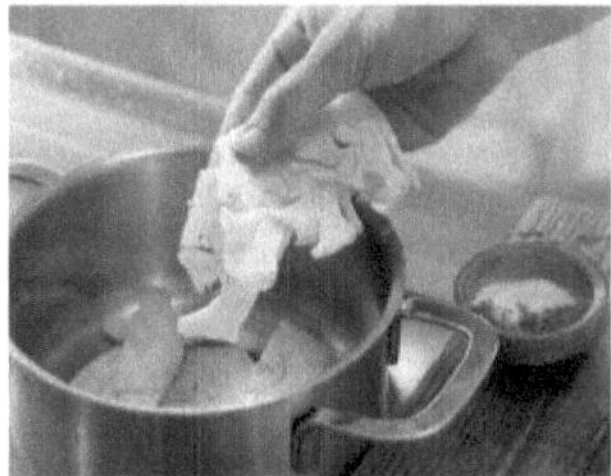

Heat 1/2 tablespoon of oil in a pot. Add the fennel, salt lightly and simmer covered over a low heat for about 2 minutes.

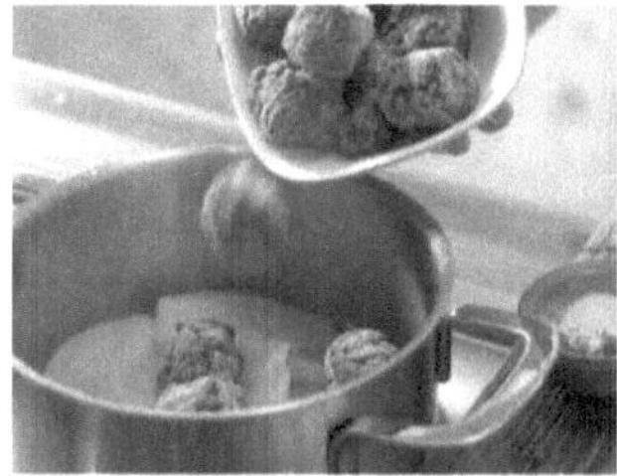

Add the leaf spinach to the fennel and cover with a lid for small Steam heat for about 5 minutes.

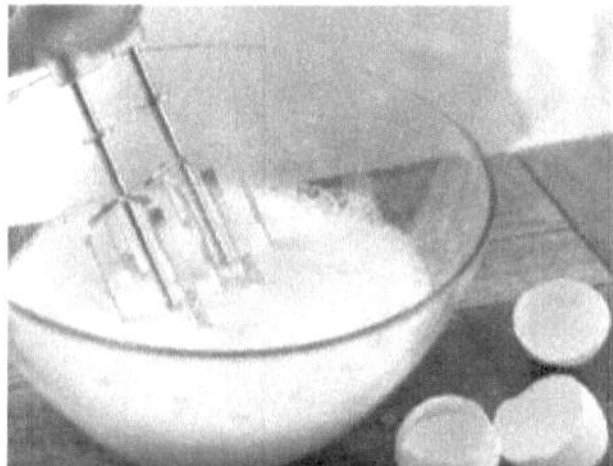

In the meantime, place the eggs and a little salt in a mixing bowl

and beat with the whisks of the hand mixer.

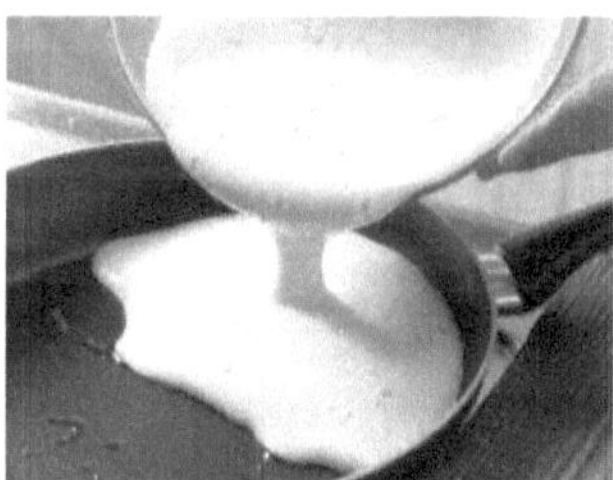

Heat the remaining oil in a coated frying pan (26 cm diameter), add the egg mixture, cover and let it simmer at low heat for about 7 minutes.

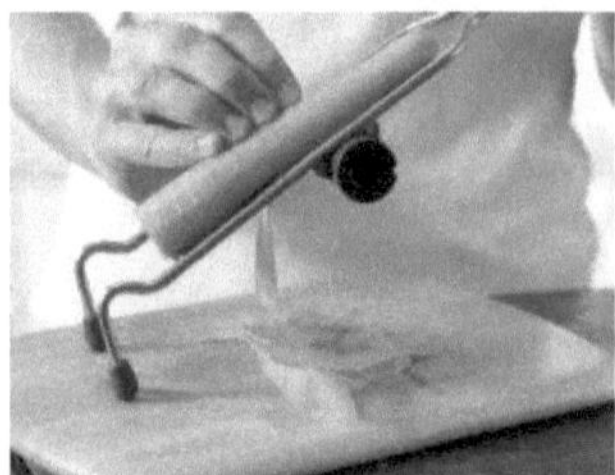

While the eggs are setting, peel the carrot, cut it into fine strips on a vegetable slicer and add it to the spinach vegetables in the pot. Season with salt and pepper and continue steaming for about 3 minutes.

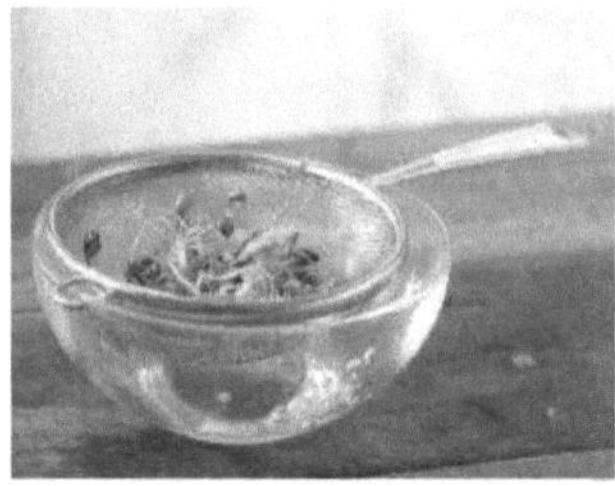

Place the sprouts in a sieve, rinse with hot water and drain.

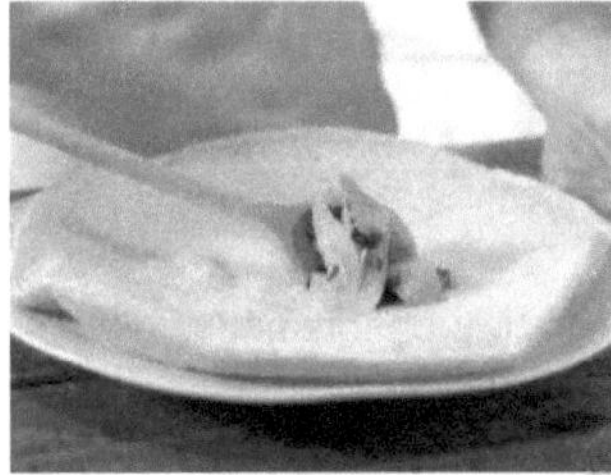

Slide the omelette onto a plate, arrange the spinach vegetables and sprouts on top. Divide into 2 halves and serve immediately.

This recipe is healthy because...

This classic from French cuisine is not only a real treat, but also a real treat: the airy omelette is bursting with vitamins, minerals and trace elements. It is particularly rich in vitamin E, which protects the cells from free radicals.

Nutritional values

1 Portion contains	(percentage of daily	requirement)
Calories	310 kcal	(15 %)
Protein	22 g	(22 %)
Fat	21 g	(18 %)
Carbohydrates	6 g	(17 %)
added sugar	0 g	(0 %)
Fibres	10 g	(33 %)

Day 5 Snack

Avocado smoothie with yoghurt and wasabi

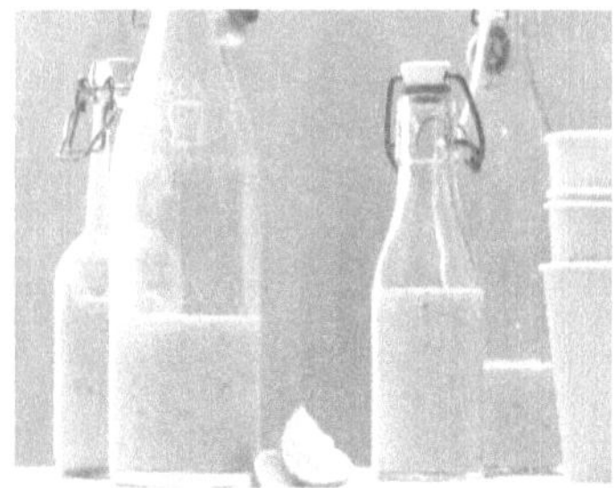

Would you like some refreshment? Then try the avocado smoothie with yoghurt and wasabi (172 calories per serving). Thanks to the avocado, this drink contains mono- and polyunsaturated fatty acids. In addition, the kefir supports the intestines in digestion. Important: Shake the avocado smoothie well before drinking!

Difficulty: easy
Preparation: 15 Minutes
Calories: 172 kcal

Ingredients for - 6 + Portions

1 bunch coriander
1 Spring onion
2 Avocados
1 Lime
1 teaspoon wasabi paste
500 ml kefir
450 g yoghurt (0,3 % fat)
2 handfuls of ice cubes
Salt
Pepper

Preparation

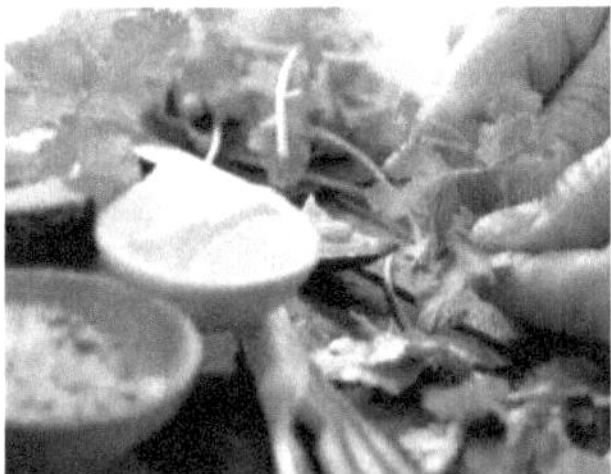

Rinse coriander, shake dry and pluck off the leaves. Clean the
spring onion, rinse, drain and cut into rings.

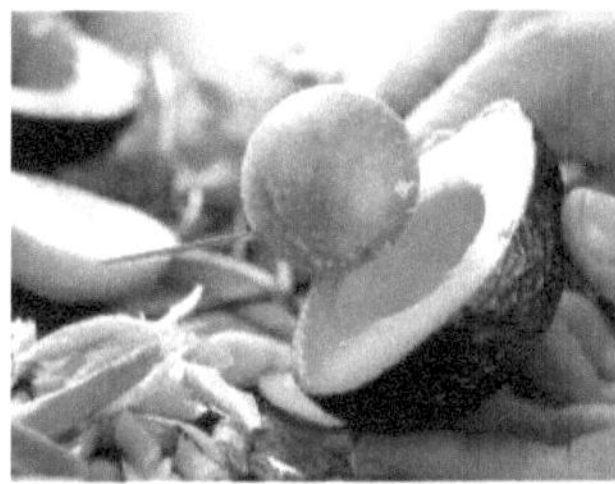

Halve and stone the avocados. Remove the flesh from the peel with a
tablespoon and place in a blender or tall container with the coriander
and spring onion rings.

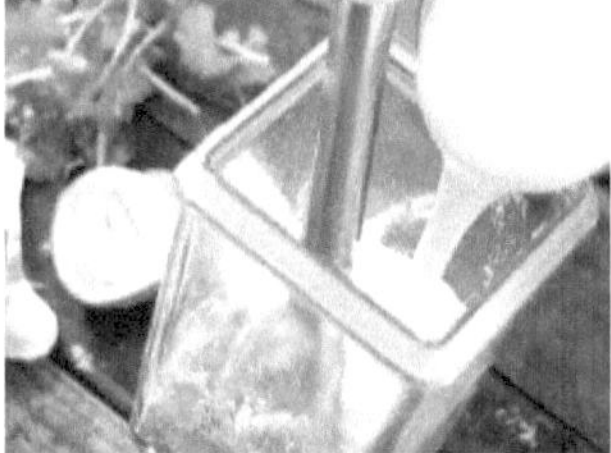

Squeeze the lime. Add 3 tablespoons of juice, wasabi paste,

kefir and yoghurt to the avocado.

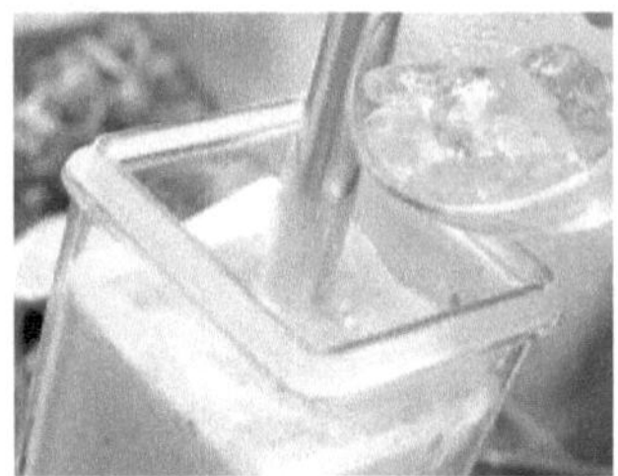

Puree everything in a mixer or with a hand blender, adding the ice cubes little by little. Season the avocado smoothie with salt and pepper and pour into glasses.

This recipe is healthy because...

If you want to save fat, you should rather do it with another ingredient: The avocado offers plenty of monounsaturated and polyunsaturated fatty acids, which have a positive influence on the cholesterol level. The sour tasting Kefir supports the intestine in its work.

Nutritional values

1 Portion contains	(percentage of daily	requirement)
Calories	172 kcal	(8 %)
Protein	7 g	(7 %)
Fat	11 g	(9 %)
Carbohydrates	7 g	(21 %)
added sugar	0 g	(0 %)
Fibres	1,5 g	(5 %)

Day 5 Lunch

Housewife-style maties in creamy sauce with onions and apples

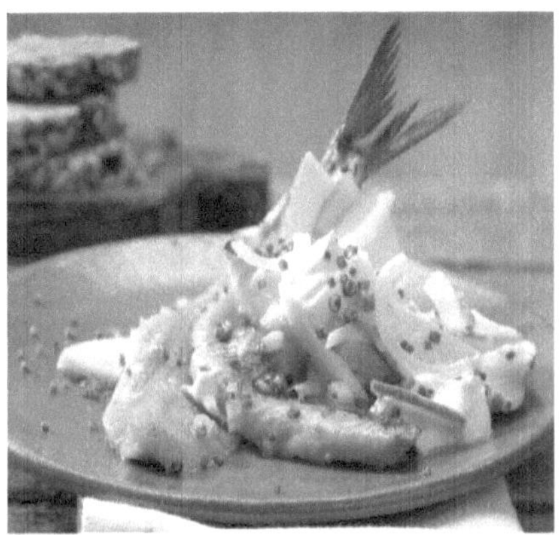

Housewife-style matjes - smarter (329 calories per serving): Lunch from the low-carb nutrition plan is on the table so easily and quickly. The classic from northern Germany scores with unsaturated fatty acids, which have a positive effect on the cholesterol level and blood lipids. Protein and B vitamins are also supplied by the matie.

<u>Difficulty:</u>   easy
<u>Preparation:</u>   20 Minutes
<u>Calories:</u>   357 kcal

Ingredients for - 4 + portions

2 small onions
2 small gherkins
2 sour apples
½ Lemon
300 g yoghurt (3,5 % fat)
Salt
Pepper
400 g double matie fillets (4 double matie fillets)
½ bunch of chives

This recipe is healthy because...

The North German classic is not low-fat, but the unsaturated fatty acids
in fish have a positive effect on blood fats and cholesterol levels. In
addition, the bones are supplied with plenty of vitamin D.

Nutritional values

1 Portion contains	(percentage of daily	requirement)
Calories	357 kcal	(17 %)
Protein	21 g	(21 %)
Fat	21 g	(18 %)
Carbohydrates	19 g	(13 %)
added sugar	0 g	(0 %)
Fibres	2,5 g	(8 %)

Preparation

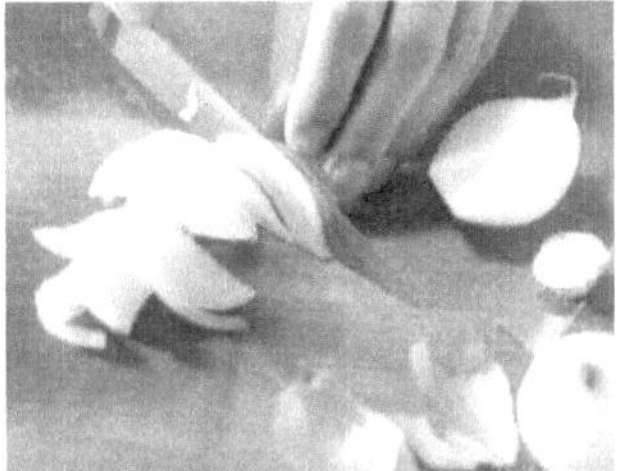

Peel onions and cut into fine strips.

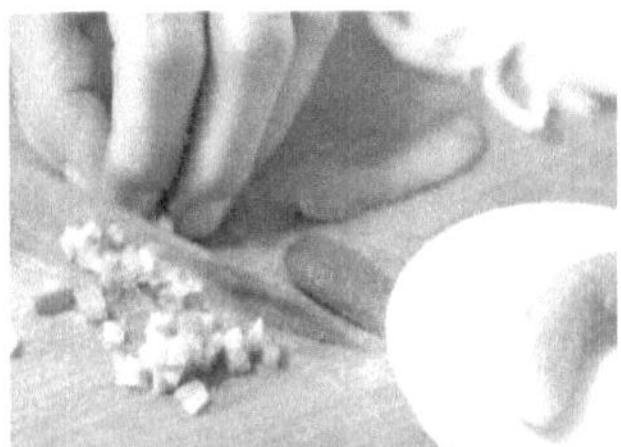

Finely dice the gherkins

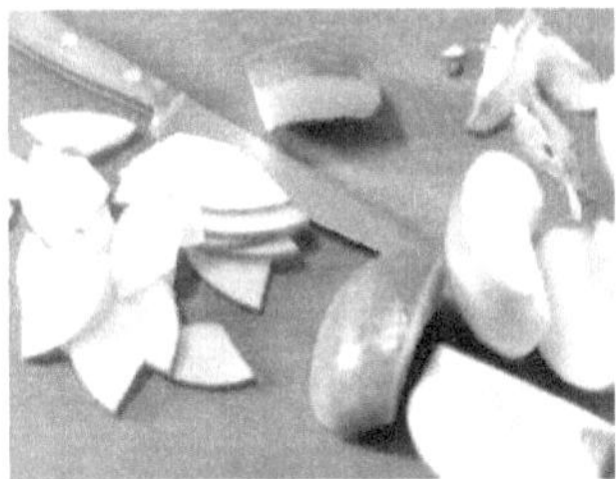

Wash and quarter the apples and remove the core. Cut the
apple quarters crosswise into thin slices. Squeeze lemon.

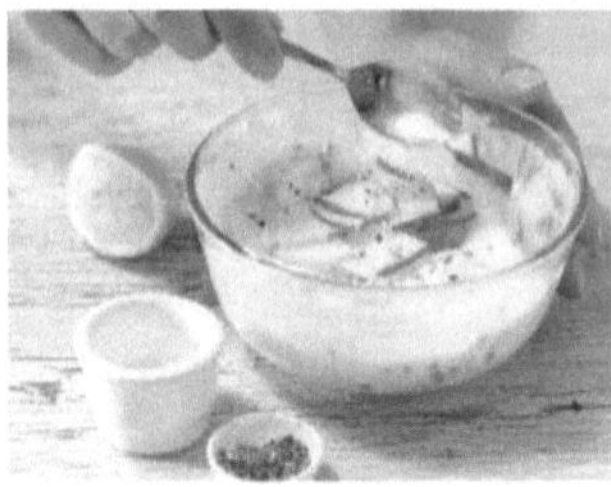

Mix yoghurt, 2 tsp. lemon juice, salt and pepper. Fold in the prepared ingredients.

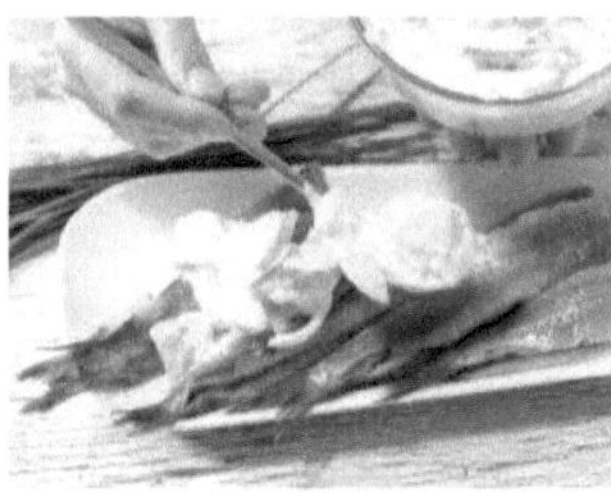

Place the matie fillets on a plate and spread the sauce over them

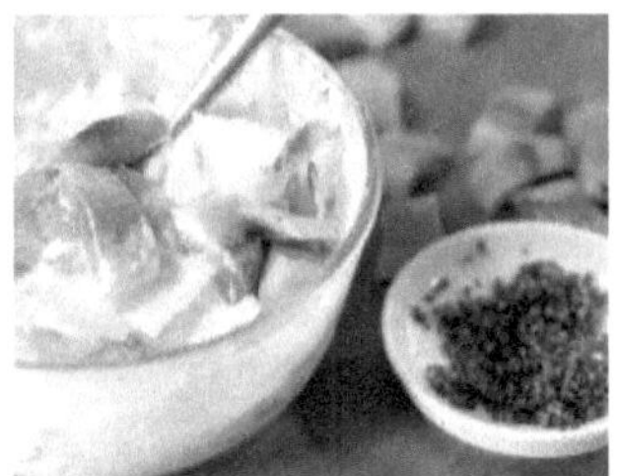

Alternatively, cut the matie fillets into small pieces and mix into the sauce. Wash the chives, shake dry, cut into fine rolls and sprinkle over the maties. Goes well with wholemeal bread.

This recipe is healthy because...

The North German classic is not low in fat, but the unsaturated fatty acids in fish have a positive effect on blood fats and cholesterol levels. In addition, the bones are supplied with plenty of vitamin D.

Nutritional values

1 Portion contains	(percentage of daily	requirement)
Calories	357 kcal	(17 %)
Protein	21 g	(21 %)
Fat	21 g	(18 %)
Carbohydrates	19 g	(13 %)
added sugar	0 g	(0 %)
Fibres	2,5 g	(8 %)

Day 6 Breakfast

Spinach salad with avocado and cress flowers

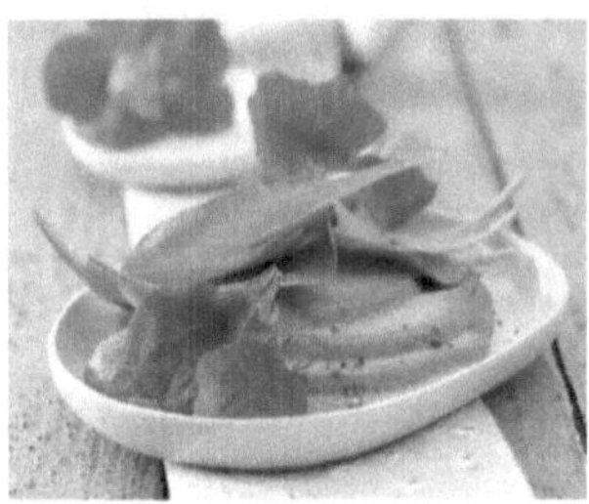

As is well known, the eye eats along - especially at this breakfast
from the low-carb nutrition plan: Spinach salad with avocado and
cress blossoms (226 calories per serving). The beautiful nasturtium
blossoms contain digestive oils as well as those that boost the
metabolism. The avocado also provides unsaturated fatty acids.

Difficulty: easy
Preparation: 25 Minutes
Calories: 226 kcal

Ingredients for – 2 + portions

150 g young leaf spinach
½ Lemon (more or less at will)
1 tablespoon elderflower syrup
Salt Pepper
1 tablespoon germ oil
175 g small ripe avocado (1 small ripe avocado)
12 Nasturtium flowers

Preparation

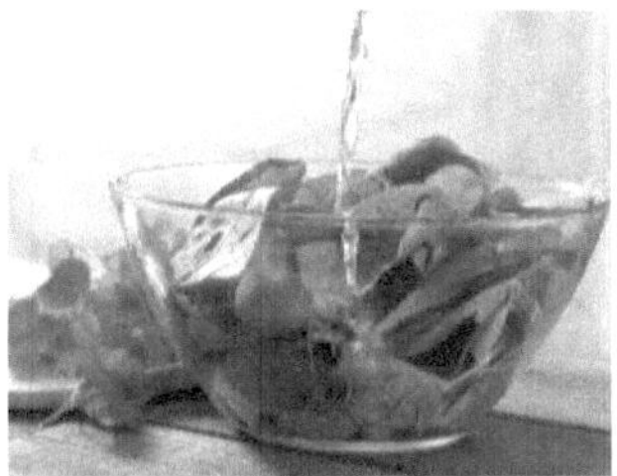

Wash spinach thoroughly, spin dry and clean.

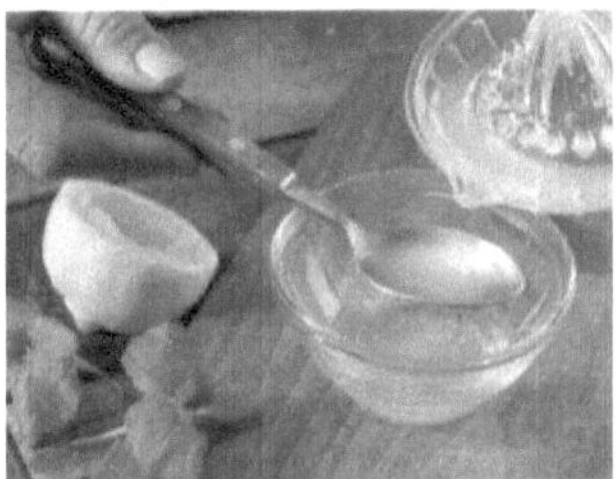

Squeeze half the lemon. Mix 2 tablespoons lemon juice with elderflower syrup, salt, pepper and oil to a salad dressing and season to taste.

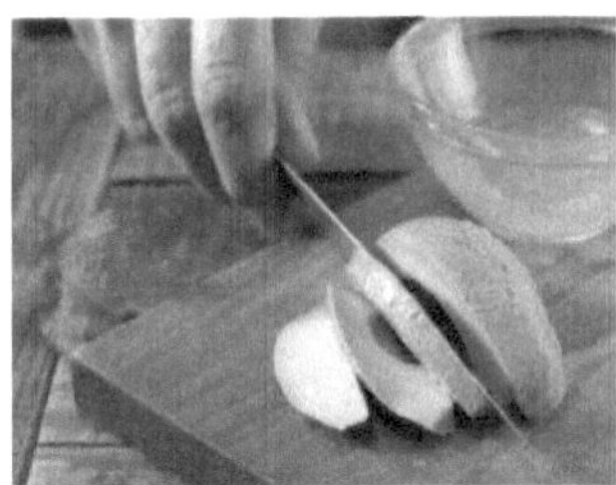

Peel and halve the avocado and remove the stone.
Cut the flesh into fine slices.

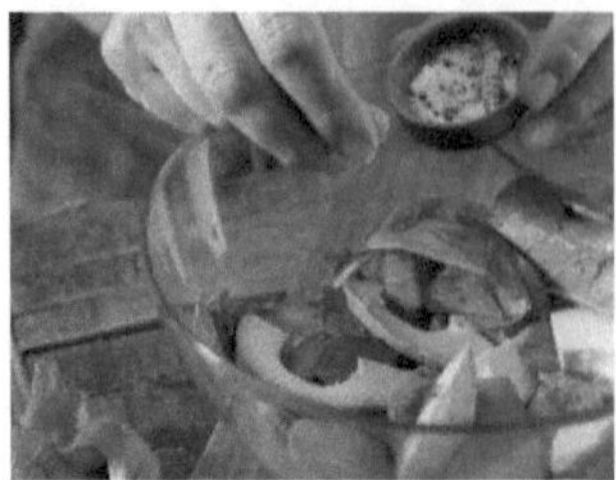

Carefully mix the avocado slices with the salad dressing. Add the spinach and carefully fold in as well. Season to taste with salt and pepper and arrange in portions.

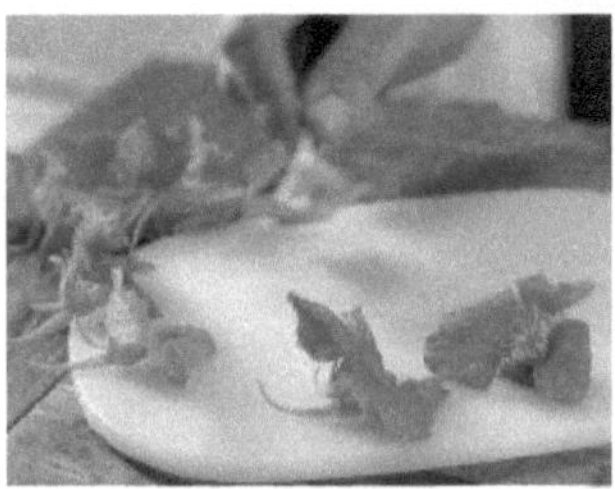

Wash the cress blossoms briefly and shake dry as desired. Garnish the spinach salad with it and serve.

This recipe is healthy because...

Don't be afraid of avocados - although they are relatively rich in fat, they provide the unsaturated fatty acids that are so valuable for the heart and blood vessels. By the way, nasturtium flowers don't just look pretty: They contain mustard oils that stimulate the metabolism and aid digestion.

Nutritional values

1 Portion contains	(percentage of daily	requirement)
Calories	226 kcal	(11 %)
Protein	3 g	(3 %)
Fat	20 g	(17 %)
Carbohydrates	6 g	(4 %)
added sugar	4 g	(16 %)
Fibres	4 g	(13 %)

Day 6 Snack

Cucumber and salmon roulade filled with cream cheese

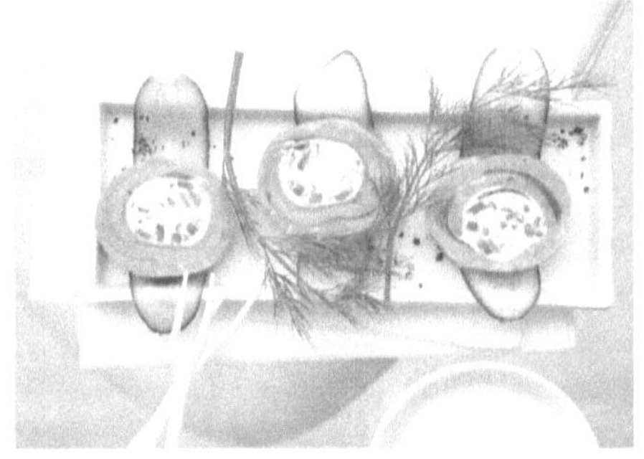

Difficulty: medium
Preparation: 45 Minutes
Calories: 98 kcal

Ingredients for - 8 + portions

2 Eggs
½ Lemon
200 g Cream cheese (13 % fat)
Salt
Pepper
1 tablespoon Worcester Sauce
2 Spring Onions
350 g large red pepper (1 large red pepper)
4 stems Dill
300 g Cucumber (1 Cucumber

Preparation

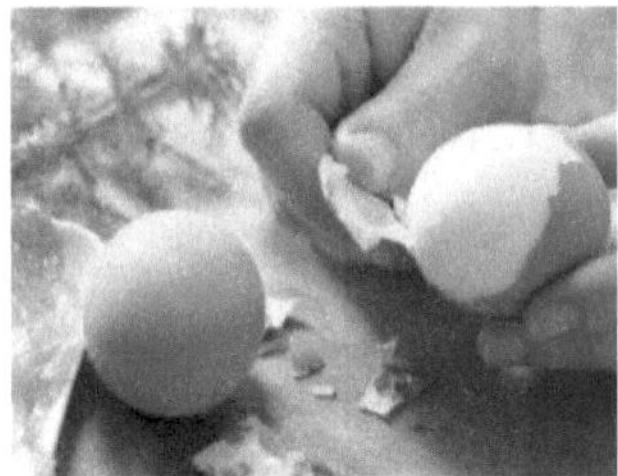

Boil eggs in boiling water for 9 minutes. Drain water, rinse eggs
with cold water and peel. Let the eggs cool down a little and then
chop them finely.

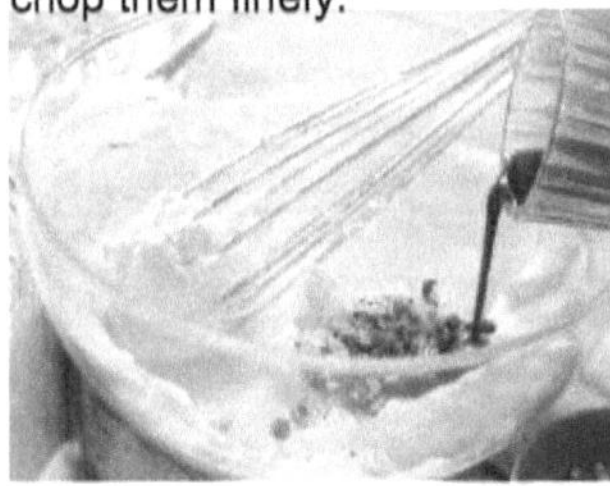

Squeeze the lemon half. Mix cream cheese in a bowl with salt,
pepper, 1 tablespoon lemon juice and Worcester sauce until
smooth.

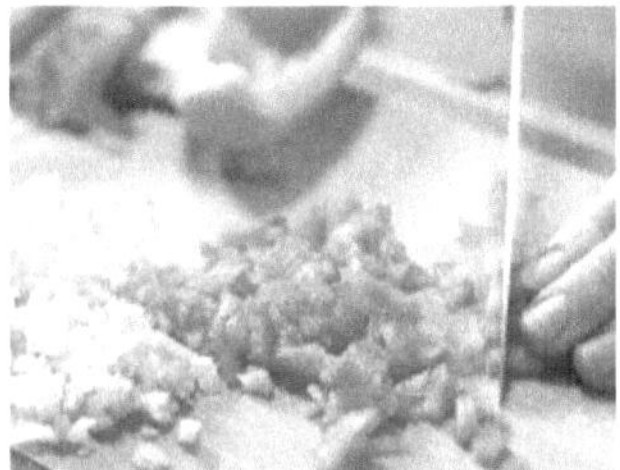

Clean and wash the spring onions and cut them into fine cubes. Cut the peppers into quarters, clean, seed, wash and finely dice them.

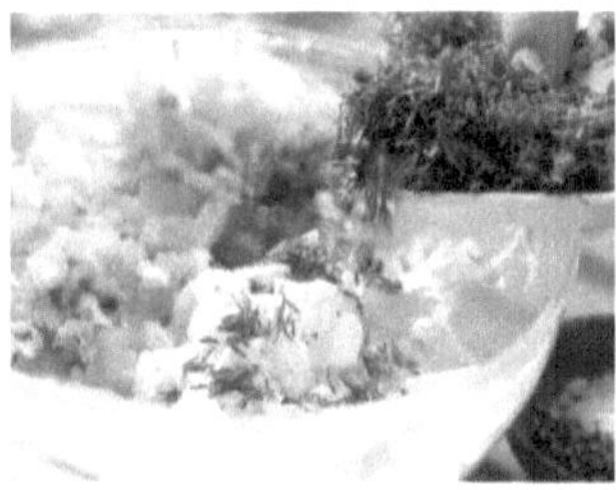

Wash the dill, shake dry, pluck the flags and cut finely. Mix eggs, spring onions, diced peppers and dill into the cheese mixture.

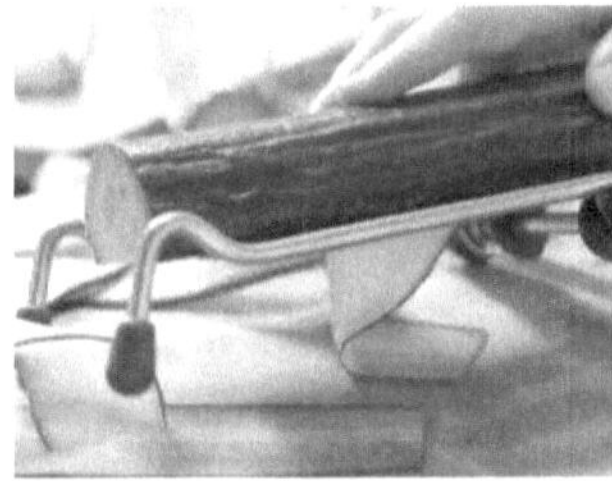

Cucumber wash, clean and cut lengthwise into thin slices. This is best done on a vegetable slicer or with a slicing machine.

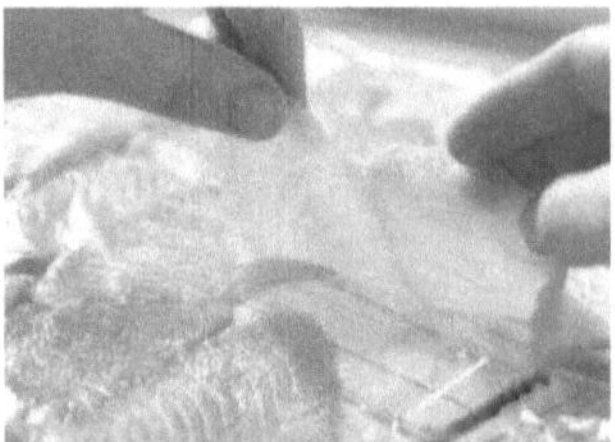

Place a piece of transparent film measuring approximately 30 x 40 cm on the work surface, overlapping the smoked salmon so that the film is almost completely covered.

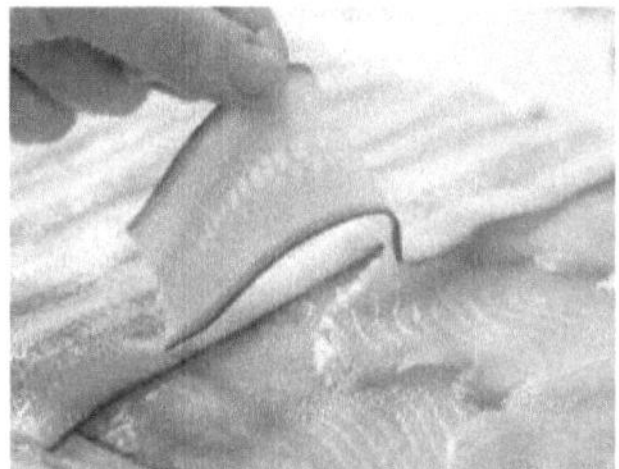

Place the cucumber slices on the salmon perpendicular to the short side of the foil overlapping (like roof tiles). Dab the cucumber slices with some kitchen paper.

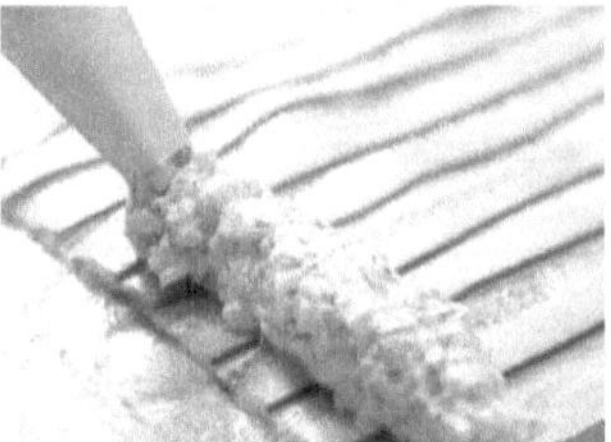

Place the cream cheese mixture in a piping bag with a piping nozzle and sharpen to the lower, short edge of the cucumber slices.

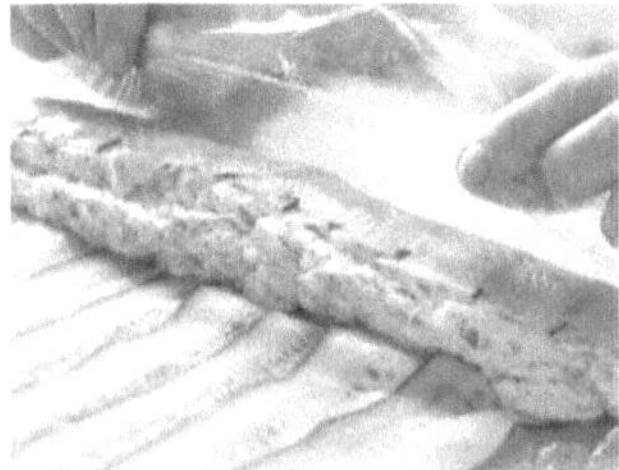

Turn the foil into a tight roll and chill for 1 hour.

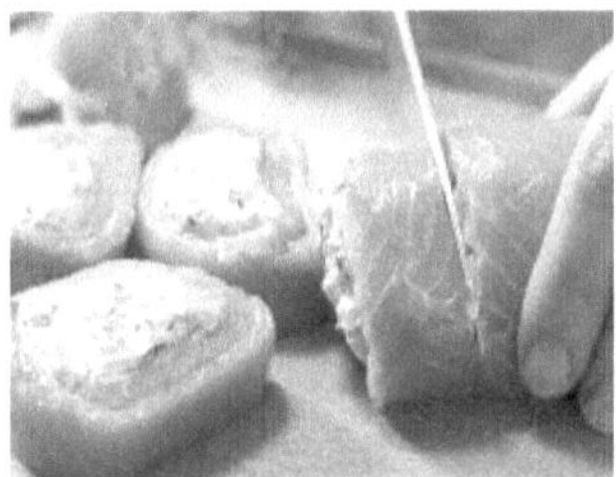

Just before serving, cut the slices into 2 cm wide pieces while still in the foil. Remove the slices from the foil and arrange them on a plate. Garnish as desired with cucumber slices and dill.

This recipe is healthy because...

The little morsels have quite a lot to offer - for example a whole day's supply of vitamin D. The fat-soluble vitamin promotes the storage of calcium and phosphate in the bones, thus ensuring their stability and resilience. Plenty of egg, cheese and fish protein as well as a dose of polyunsaturated fatty acids (good for the heart and circulation!) from salmon increase the benefits.

Nutritional values

1 Portion contains	(percentage of daily	requirement)
Calories	98 kcal	(5 %)
Protein	9 g	(9 %)
Fat	5 g	(4 %)
Carbohydrates	3 g	(2 %)
added sugar	0 g	(0 %)
Fibres	2 g	(7 %)

Day 6 Lunch

Tatar meatballs with tomato and olive salad

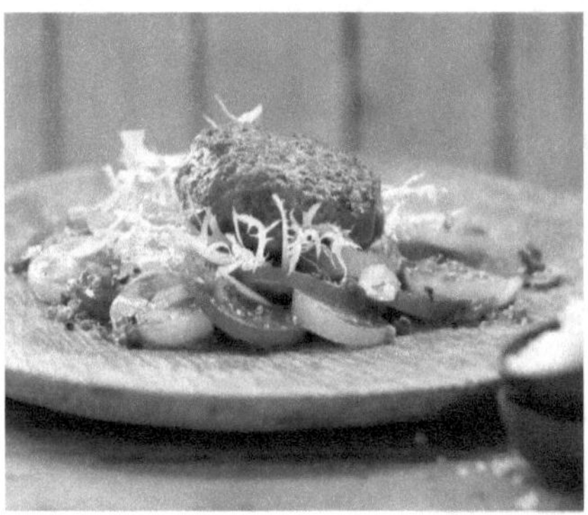

In a quick 30 minutes this lunch is on the table: Tatar meatballs with tomato and olive salad (339 calories per portion). The beef tartar is prepared from lean beefsteak, provides iron and vitamin B12 - of course, a large portion of the satiating protein is also included.

Difficulty: easy
Preparation: 30 Minutes
Calories: 339 kcal

Ingredients for - 4 +portions

1 Onion
400 g Beef Tatar
2 egg yolk
½ tsp. Dijon mustard
Salt
Pepper
1 tsp. Ketchup
1 tsp. Worcester sauce
400 g Tomatoes (red and yellow, 8 tomatoes)
100 g Frisée salad (half a frisée salad)
75 g green olives with stone
½ bunch chives
4 tsp Olive oil
1 tsp Balsamic vinegar
cane sugar

Prepartion

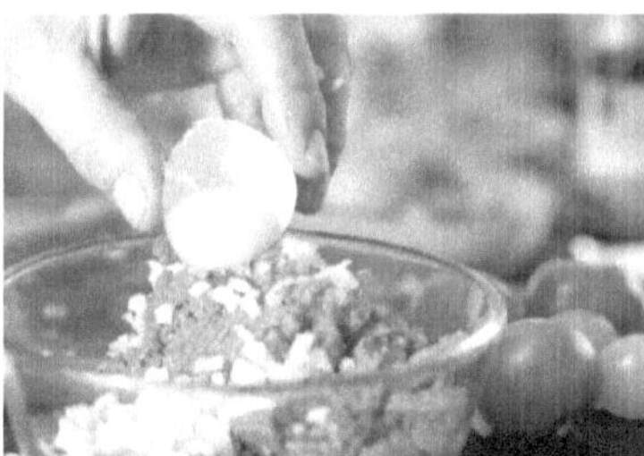

Peel and finely chop the onion. Separate the eggs (use the egg whites for other purposes). Mix shallot with tartar, egg yolks, mustard, ketchup, salt and pepper.

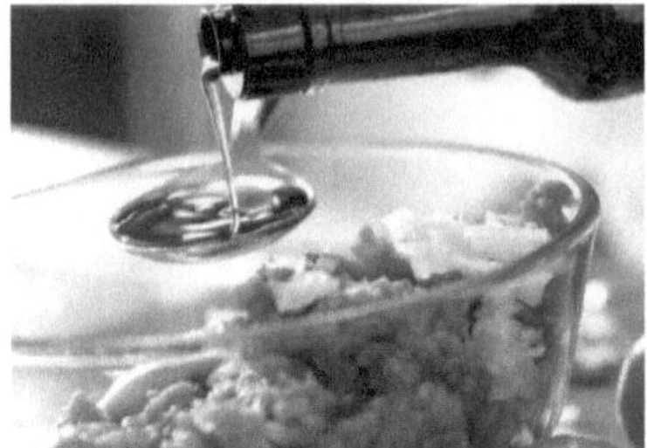

Add the Worcester sauce.

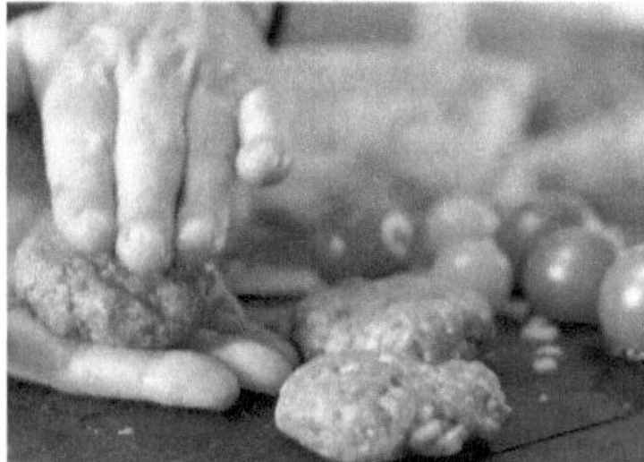

Shape into 4 meatballs with damp hands and chill.

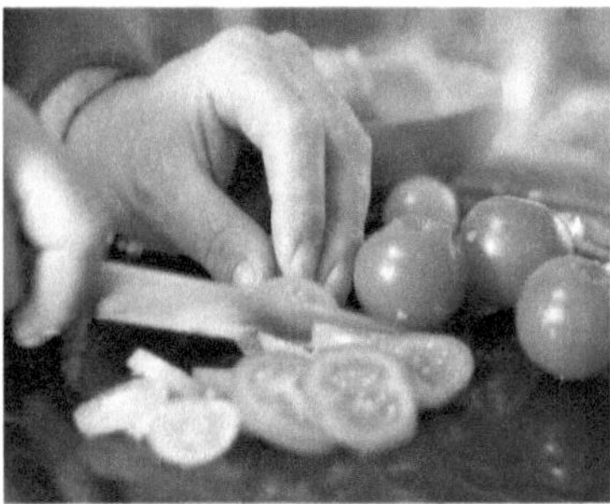

Wash 4 tomatoes, cut out the stalks in a wedge shape and slice the tomatoes.

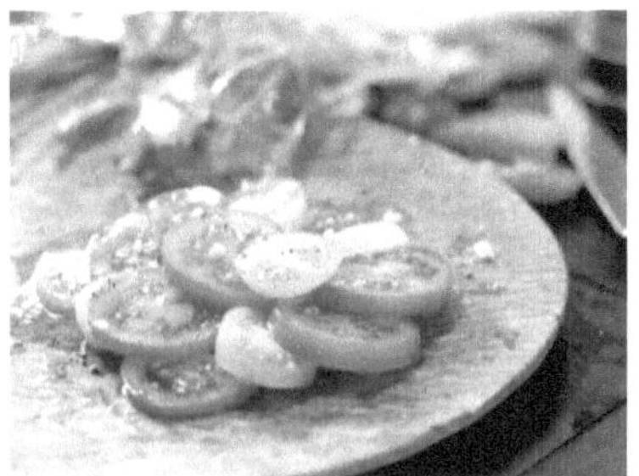

Place tomato slices decoratively on plates and season with salt and pepper.

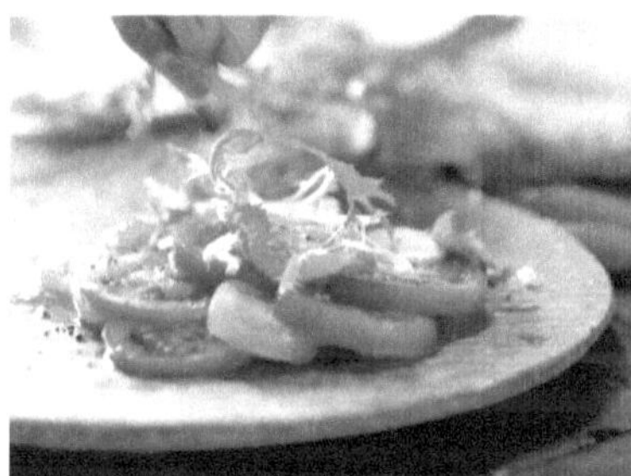

Clean, wash and spin-dry frisée lettuce and divide into bite-sized pieces. Spread on the tomatoes.

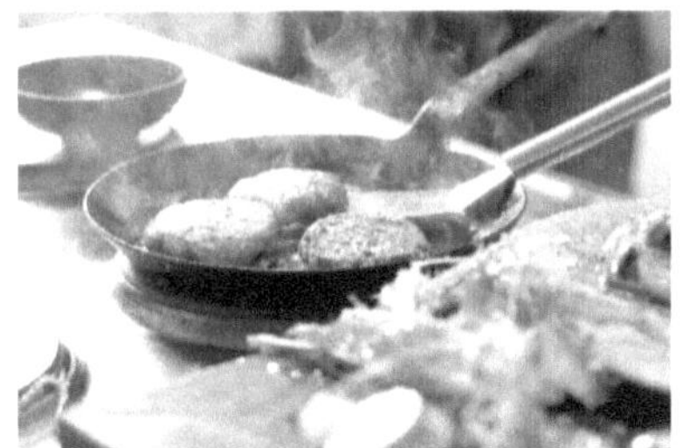

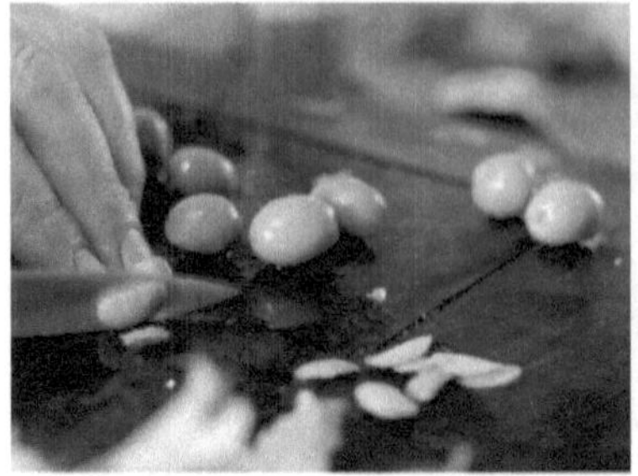

Cut olives in thin slices from the stone.

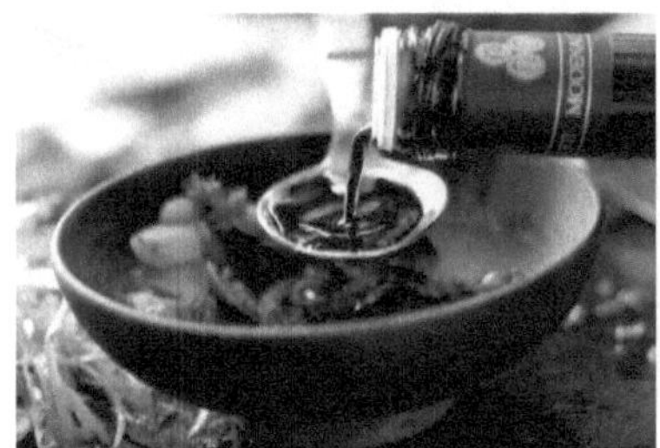

Cut the chives into fine rolls. Mix with olives, 3 tablespoons olive oil, vinegar and 1 pinch of sugar.

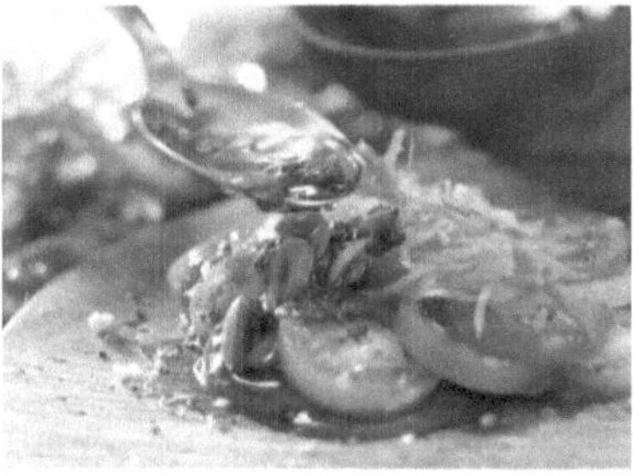

Pour over the tomatoes.

Heat a heavy pan and add the remaining oil. Place the tartar meatballs in it and fry on each side for 20 seconds over a very high heat. Remove meat from the pan with a spatula or pallet. Serve the tartar meatballs with the tomatoes.

Day 6 Evening meal

Goulash soup with peppers and potatoes

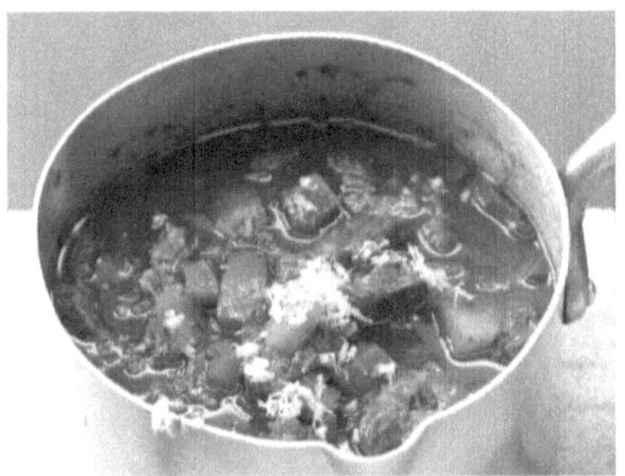

This goulash soup (234 calories per portion) is not only smarter, it can be prepared in large quantities and then frozen. So there is always a portion of the low-carb soup classic in the cooler as a reserve. The meat contains protein, the vegetables provide vitamins and fibre - a perfect combination!

Difficulty: easy
Prepariton: 1 h 10 Minutes

Ingredients for- 4 + portions

300 g beef (from the topside or rump)
1 large red onion
1 red pepper
1 yellow pepper
2 tablespoons rapeseed oil
2 tablespoons tomato paste
1 tablespoon paprika powder (sweet)
1 tablespoon paprika powder (rose hot)
200 ml dry red wine
600 ml classic vegetable broth
200 g potatoes
1 small organic lemon
1 garlic clove
1 tsp caraway
Salt
Parsley (at will)

Preparation

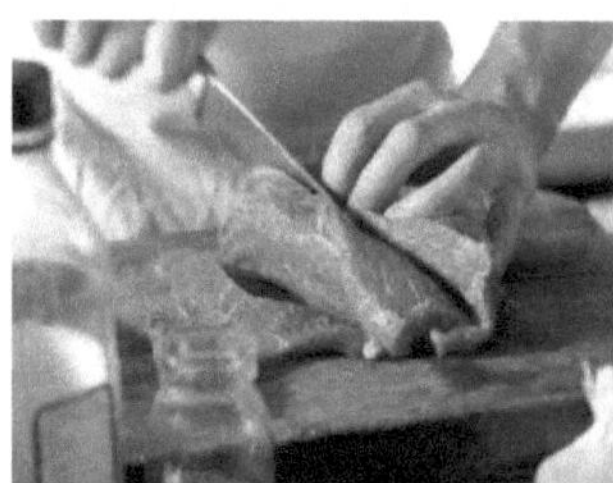

Dab meat dry and cut into small cubes.

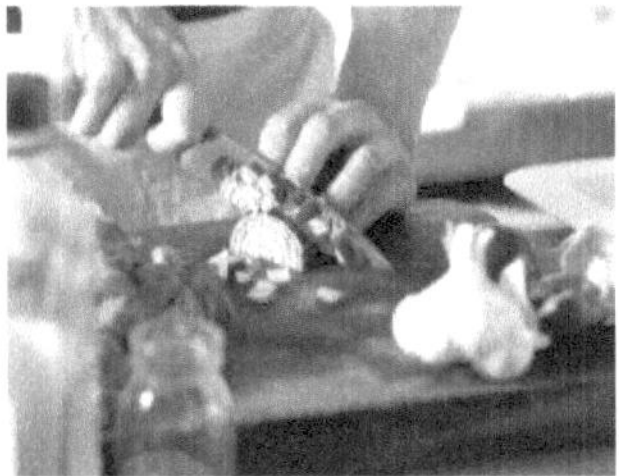

Peel onion and cut into fine cubes.

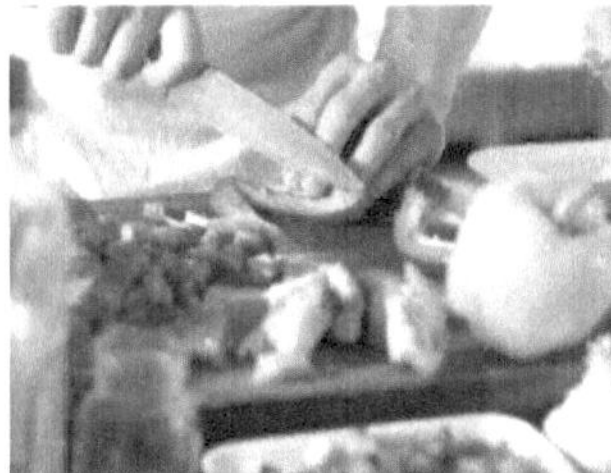

Cut the peppers into quarters, clean, seed, wash and also cut into cubes.

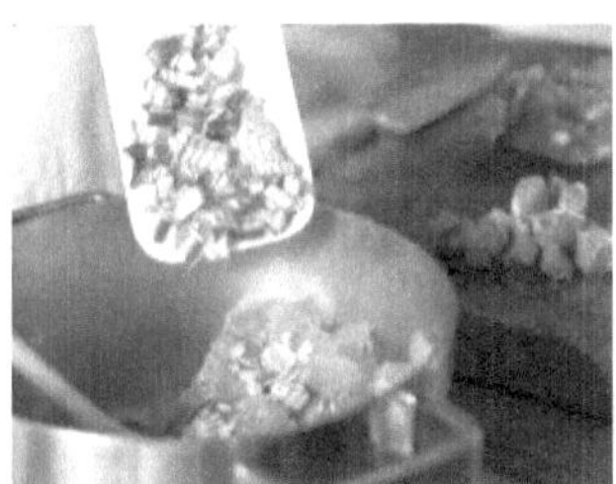

Heat the oil in a pot, fry the onion cubes and meat well.

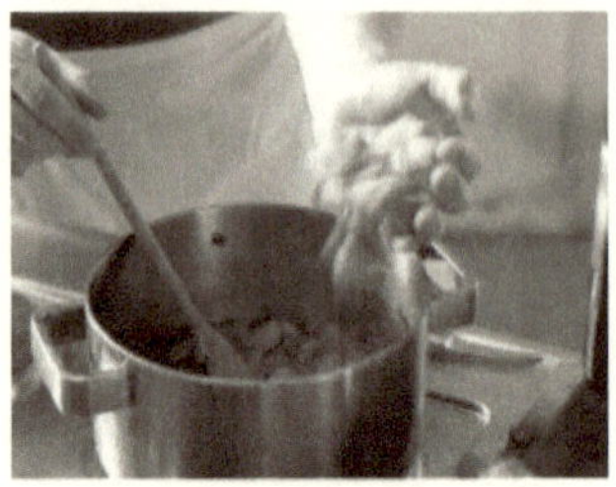

Add the diced peppers and fry for 1 minute.

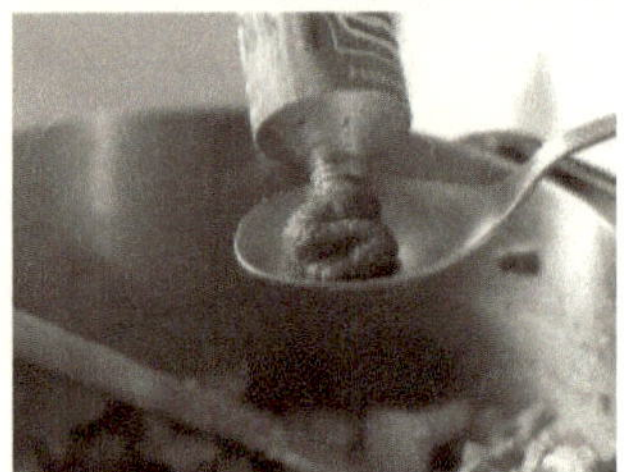

Add tomato paste and paprika powder and mix everything well.

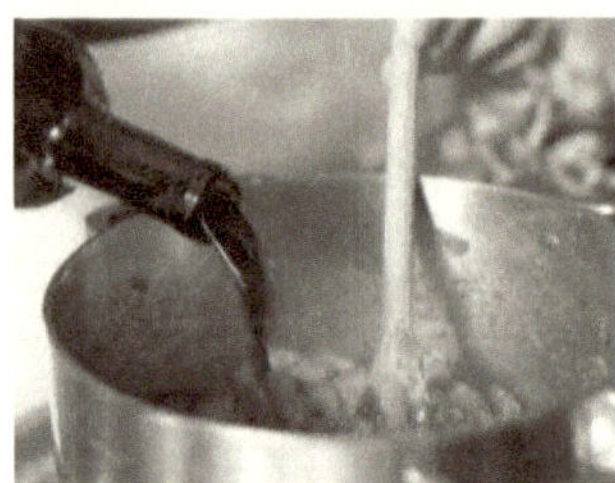

Add red wine and broth and bring everything to the boil.

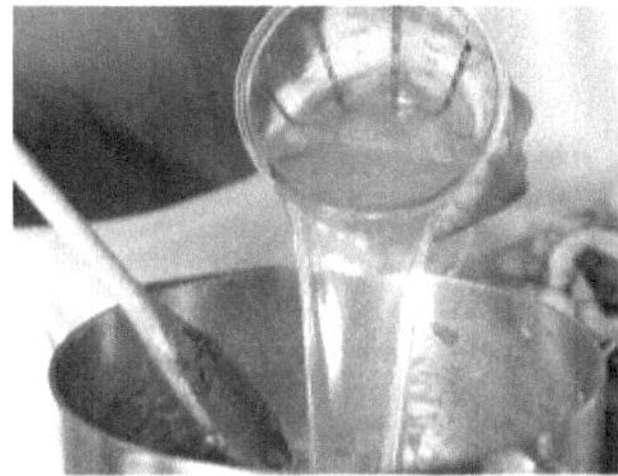

Cook the goulash at medium heat for 20 to 30 minutes.

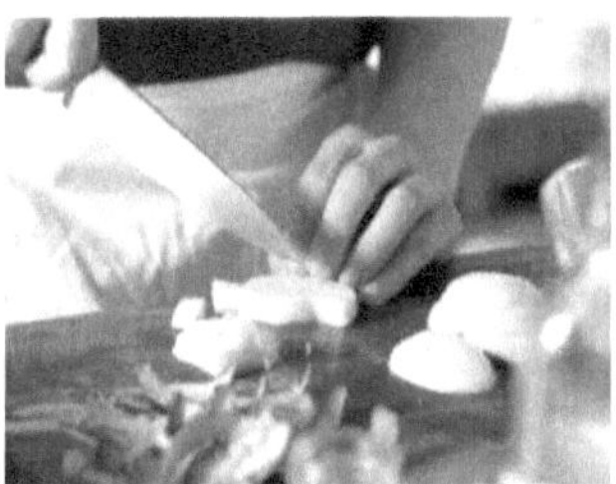

Wash and peel the potatoes and cut them into 1 cm cubes. Add the potatoes to the pot, bring everything to the boil again and cook for another 25 minutes. Rinse lemon hot, dry and grate half of the peel finely. Peel garlic, chop together with lemon peel, caraway and 1 pinch of salt. Add to the goulash soup 5 minutes before the end of cooking time. Sprinkle goulash soup with some chopped parsley and lemon peel before serving.

This recipe is healthy because...

This light goulash soup has earned the green Mandelbrot-Set in the Health Score: the meat provides a lot of protein, the vegetables the necessary dietary fibre. Compared to vegetable iron, the iron contained in beef can be easily absorbed by the body. We need this mineral for healthy blood formation and oxygen transport in the blood.

Nutritional values

1 Portion contains	(percentage of daily	requirement)
Calories	234 kcal	(11 %)
Protein	24 g	(24 %)
Fat	9 g	(8 %)
Carbohydrates	11 g	(7 %)
added sugar	0 g	(0 %)
Fibres	5,5 g	(18 %)

Day 7 Breakfast

Asian scrambled eggs with bean sprouts

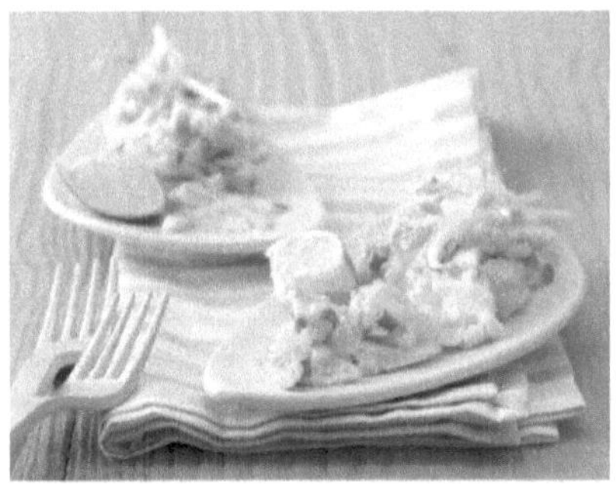

Asian scrambled eggs with bean sprouts (200 calories per serving) are served. In only 20 minutes, the filling breakfast is on the table and provides, besides protein, half the daily requirement of vitamin D. The bean sprouts ensure a crunchy bite in the scrambled eggs.

<u>Difficulty:</u> easy
<u>Preparation:</u> 20 Minutes
<u>Calories:</u> 200 kcal

Ingredients for - 2 + portions

20 g ginger (1 piece)
½ bunch of spring onions
½ red chilli pepper
½ Stick of lemongrass
3 eggs
3 tablespoons coconut milk (9% fat) Salt
100 g sprouts (e.g. bean sprouts)
½ Lime

Preparation

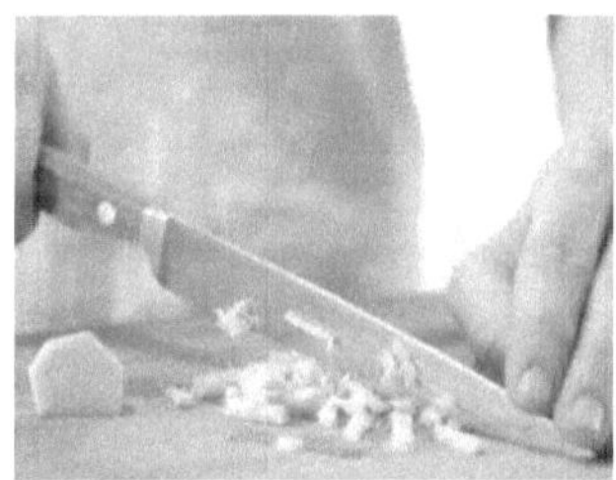

Peel and finely chop the ginger.

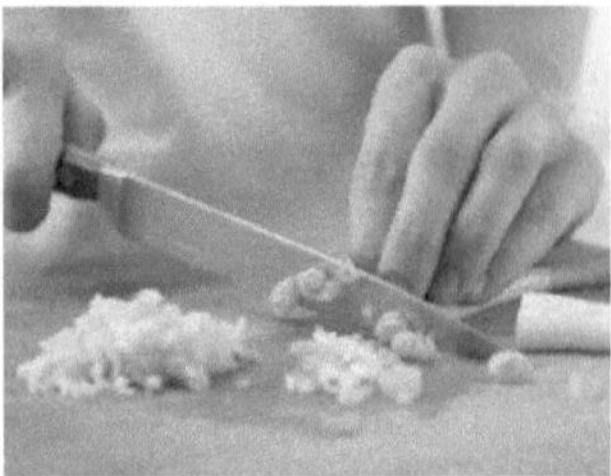

Clean and wash the spring onions and cut them into fine
rings.

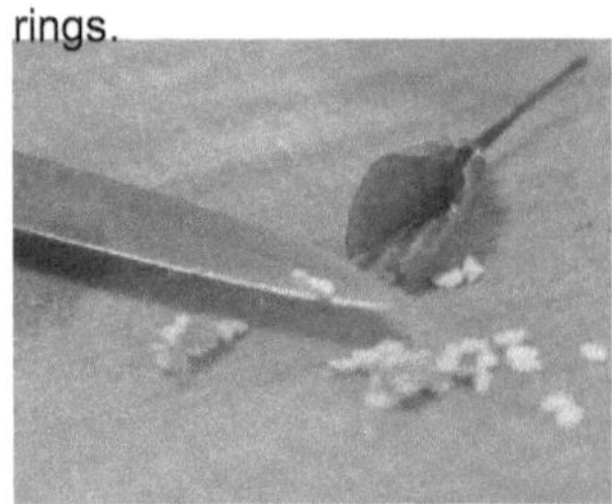

Halve the chili pepper lengthwise, remove seeds, wash and chop
finely.

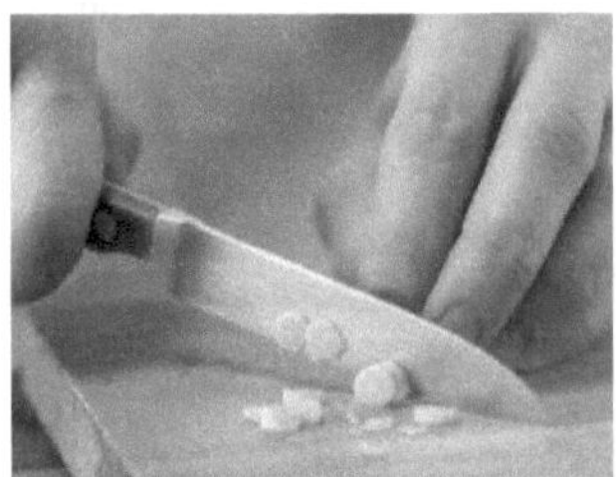

If present, remove the hard outer leaves from the lemon grass
and cut off the root base. Finely chop the bottom 5 cm of the
stem.

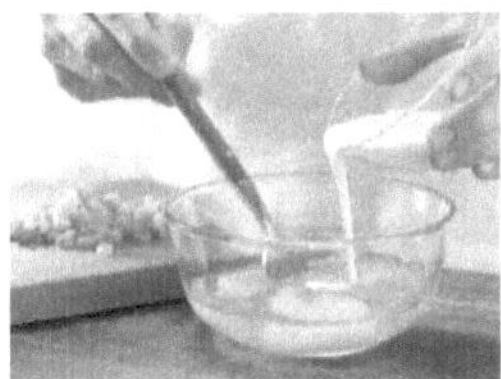

Whisk eggs and coconut milk. Season with salt. Stir in ginger, spring onions, chili and lemongrass.

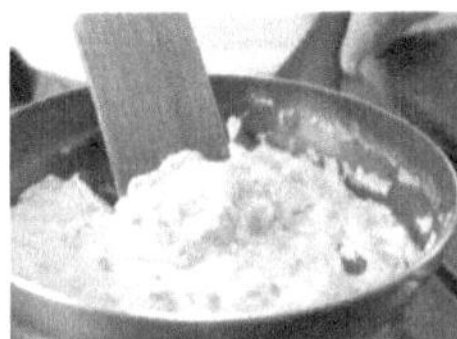

Pour the egg mixture into a coated pan and allow it to set (set) over a low heat, using a spatula to draw several times through the egg mixture from the edge of the pan to the middle.

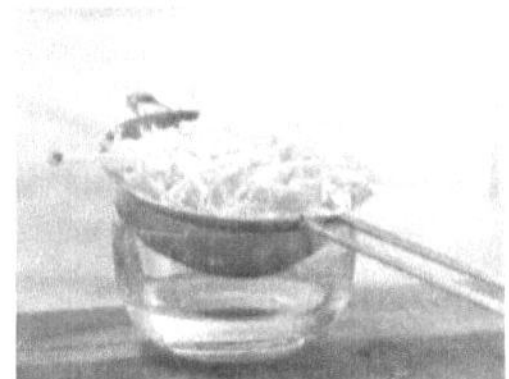

Put the sprouts in a sieve, rinse and drain well.

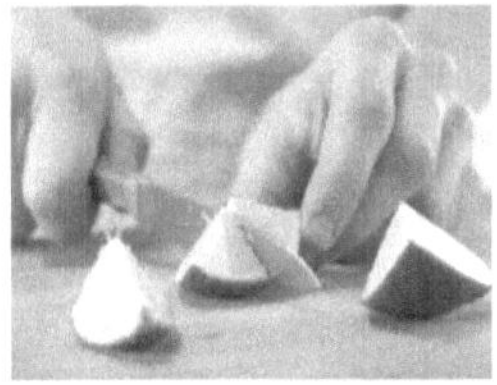

Rinse the lime half hot and cut into slices or pieces.
Arrange scrambled eggs with sprouts and lime wedges.

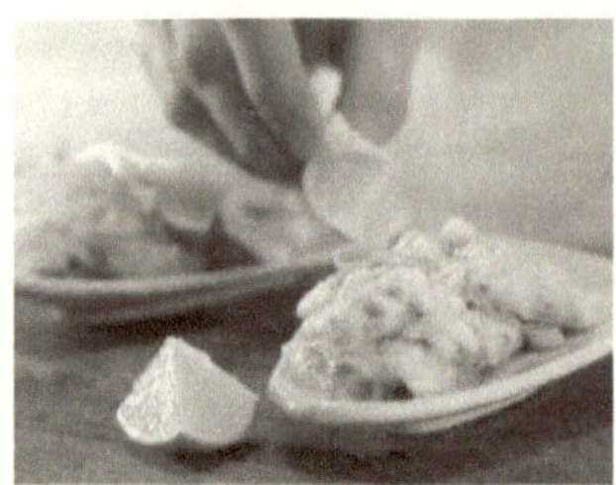

This recipe is healthy because...

The high-protein meal is perfect for a light dinner or brunch. In addition to half the daily requirement of vitamin D, one portion contains 40 percent pantothenic acid. Diabetics and dialysis patients in particular should keep an eye on the supply of this substance, which is one of the B vitamins - as should anyone who regularly drinks alcohol.

Nutritional values

1 Portion contains	(percentage of daily	requirement)
Calories	200 kcal	(10 %)
Protein	15 g	(15 %)
Fat	12 g	(10 %)
Carbohydrates	7 g	(5 %)
added sugar	0 g	(0 %)
Fibres	2 g	(7 %)

Day 7 Snack

Pecorino cheese skewers with spice-herb-oil

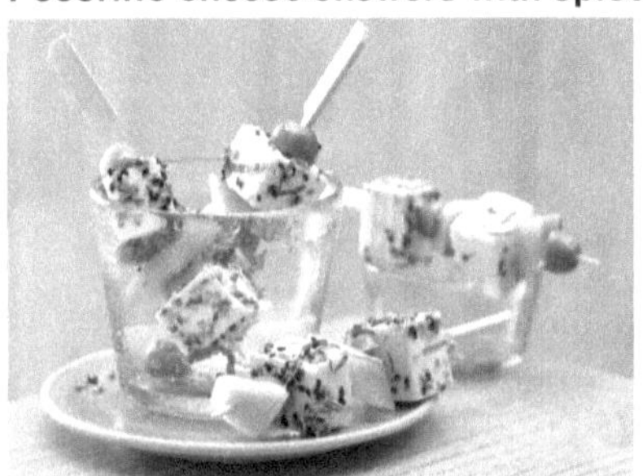

Protein on the skewers is provided by the sheep's cheese skewers with spiced herb oil (66 calories per portion). Pecorino cheese supplies the body with calcium, which is important for bones and teeth. Mini tomatoes make this skewer even more fruity!

Difficulty: easy
Preparation: 30 Minutes
Calories: 66 kcal

Ingredients for – 10 + skewers

1 tablespoon light sesam
1 tablespoon black sesame
1 tablespoon fennel seed
200 g Pecorino cheese (9 % fat absolute)
1 Organic lemon
2 tablespoon of olive oil
salt
1 tablespoon coarsely ground black pepper
4 stems mint
200 g cucumber (half a cucumber)
10 green olives (without stone)

Preparation

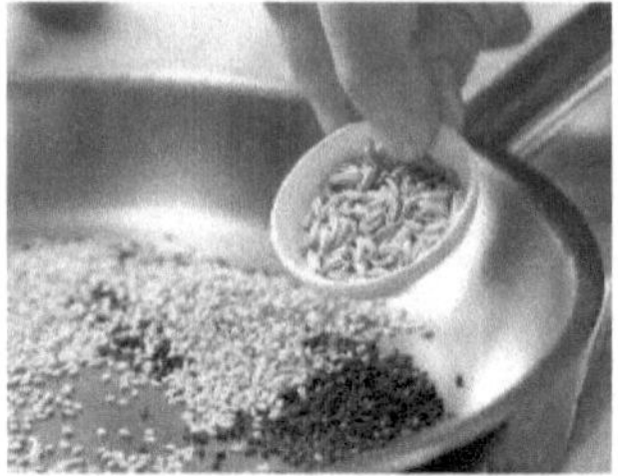

Roast the sesame and fennel seeds in a coated pan without fat and allow to cool.

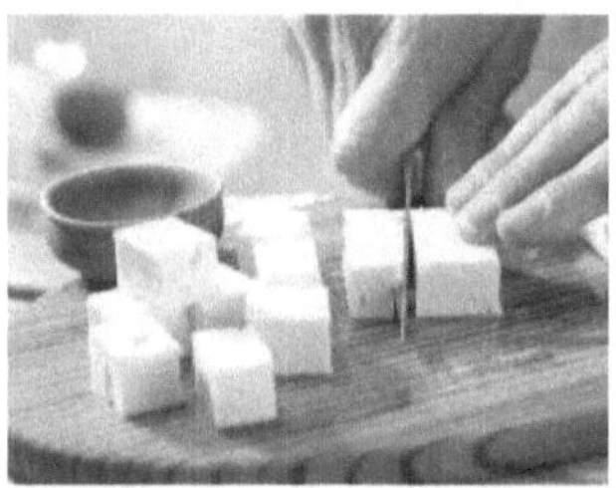

Drain the feta cheese and cut into 20 cubes of about the same size.

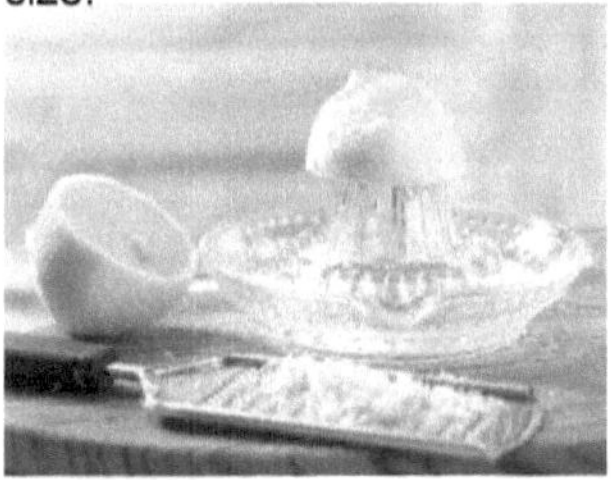

Rinse lemon hot, rub dry and finely grate the peel. Squeeze one half of the lemon (use the rest for other purposes) and measure 1 tbsp. juice.

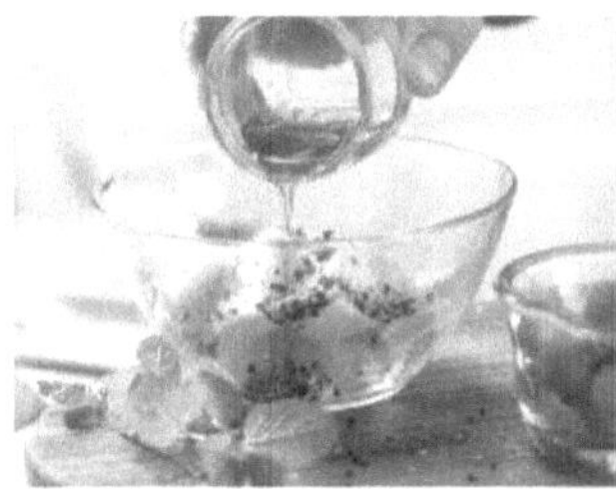

Mix fennel seed, sesame, lemon juice, lemon peel, oil, 1 pinch of salt
and pepper in a bowl. Turn the diced feta cheese in it, cover and put
it in the refrigerator for 4 hours (marinate).

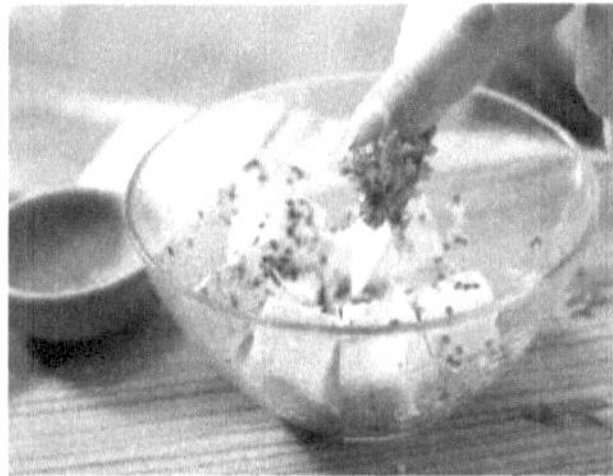

Wash mint, shake dry, pluck off leaves, chop finely and mix with
the cheese cubes.

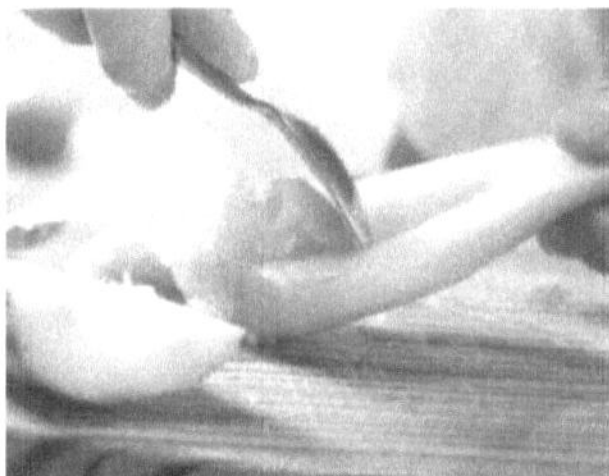

Peel half the cucumber, cut it in half and remove the seeds
with a spoon. Cut the cucumber into cubes of about 1 cm.

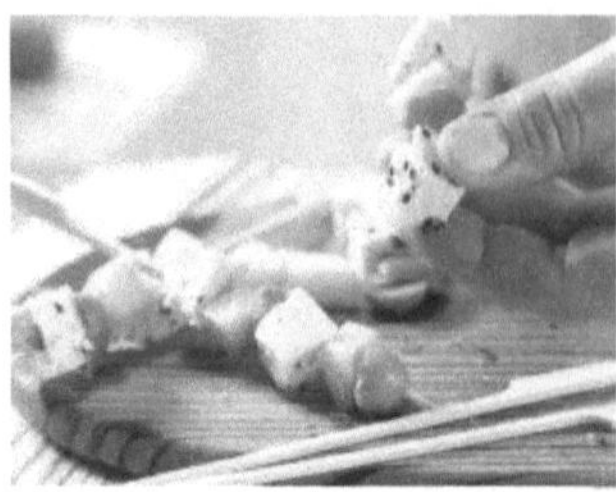

Drain the olives in a small sieve and cut them in half. Alternately put cucumber and cheese cubes on 10 skewers and serve..

This recipe is healthy because...

Pecorino cheese provides the body with valuable calcium. The mineral not only ensures healthy bones and teeth, but also helps to heal wounds and is involved in blood clotting.

Nutritional values

1 Skewer contains	(percentage of daily	requirement)
Calories	66 kcal	(3 %)
Protein	2 g	(2 %)
Fat	6 g	(5 %)
Carbohydrates	1 g	(1 %)
added sugar	0 g	(0 %)
Fibres	0,5 g	(2 %)

Day 7 Lunch

Turkey braised with ratatouille vegetables

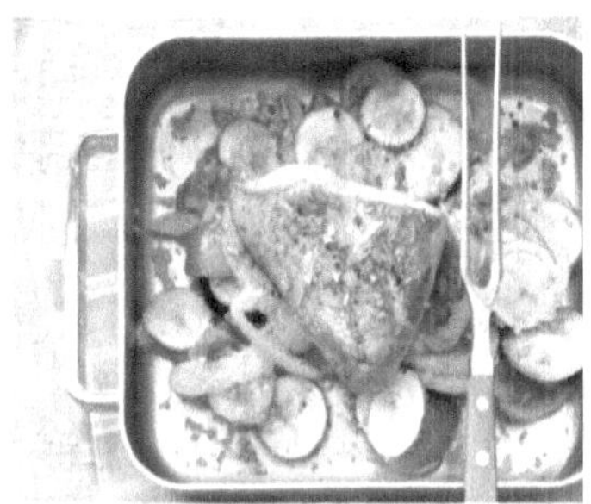

Turkey braised with ratatouille vegetables (433 calories per serving) is on the low-carb diet for lunch. Although the spicy braised turkey takes about an hour to prepare, its ingredients are worth the wait. The colourful mixture of vegetables provides vitamins, minerals and fibre. The lean turkey meat scores with a low fat content and high-quality protein.

Difficulty: medium
Preparation: 30 Minutes
Calories: 433 kcal

Ingredients for - 2 + portions

500 g turkey breast fillet
2 tablespoons rapeseed oil
100 ml classic vegetable broth
½ Covenant Tarragon
Salt
Pepper
1 garlic clove
2 onions
1 small yellow pepper

1 sprig of thyme
½ small zucchini
2 tomatoes
1 lemon
½ small aubergine

Preparation

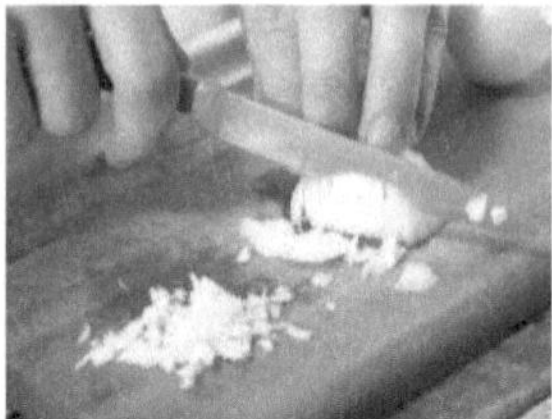

Rinse turkey breast, dab dry, salt and pepper. Peel and chop the garlic
and onions.

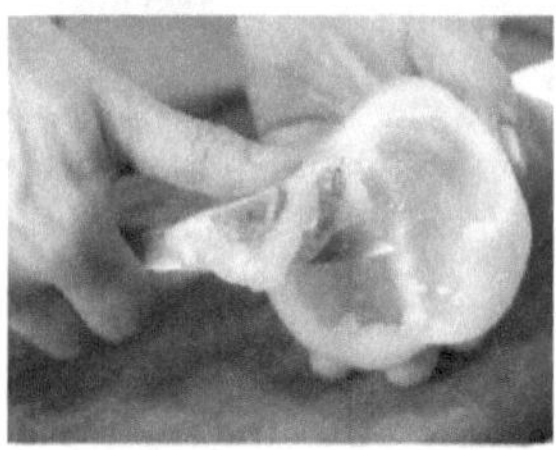

Halve the pepper, remove seeds, wash and cut into fine strips.

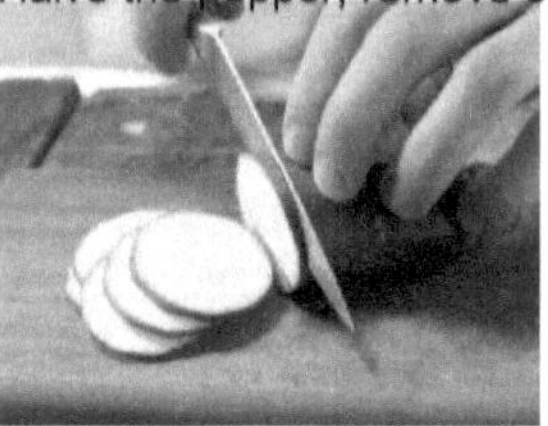

Wash aubergine and zucchini and cut into thin slices.

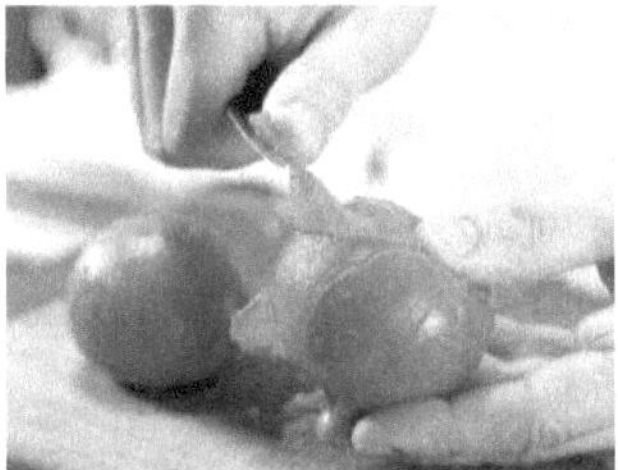

Dip tomatoes briefly in boiling water, remove, rinse cold and peel the skin.

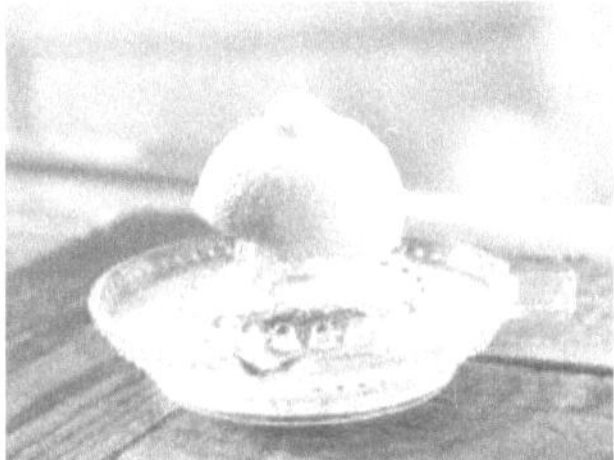

Halve the lemon and squeeze the juice.

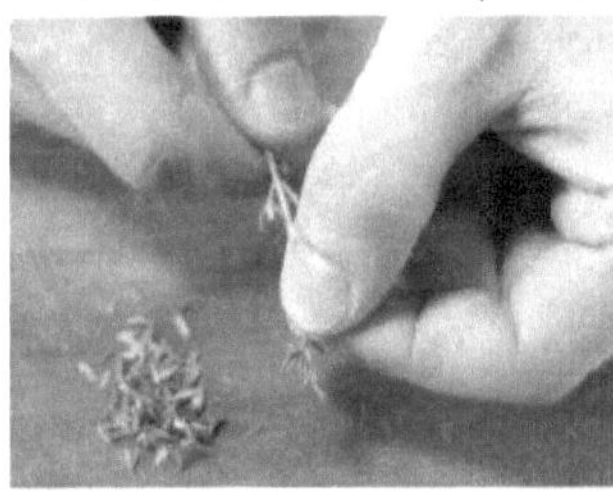

Rinse the thyme, shake dry and pluck the leaves.

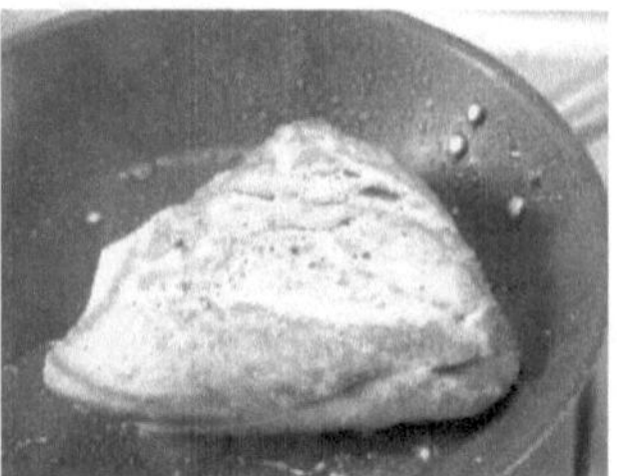

Heat 1 tablespoon of oil in a coated frying pan. Brown the turkey breast in it all around at medium heat, take it out and put it aside on a plate.

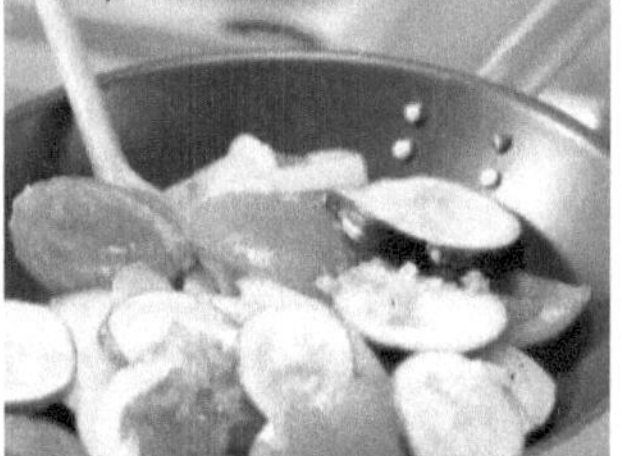

Add the remaining oil to the pan. Sauté the onions and garlic until transparent. Add the pepper strips, aubergines, zucchini and tomatoes and steam for about 2 minutes while stirring.

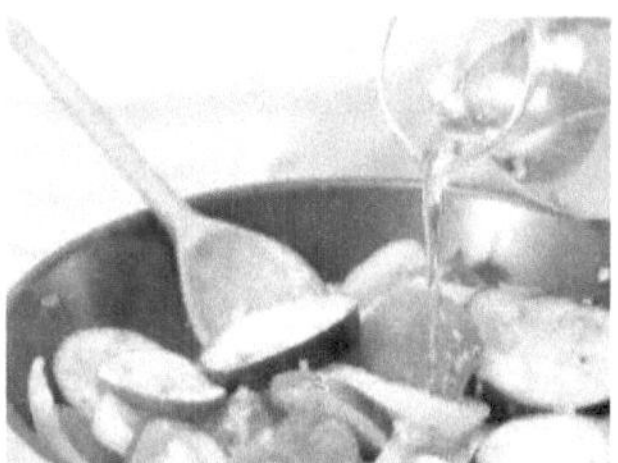

Stir in thyme, lemon juice and vegetable stock and cook over medium heat for 10 to12 minutes, stirring occasionally. Then place in a small roaster.

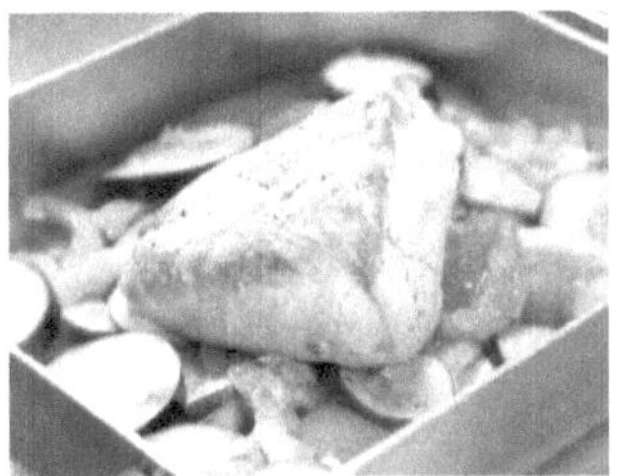

Place the turkey breast on top and braise covered in a preheated oven at 200 °C (fan oven: 180 °C, gas: level 4) for about 30 minutes.

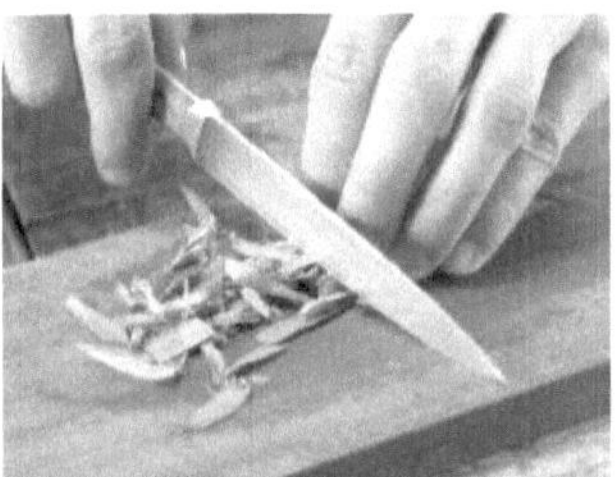

Meanwhile, wash the tarragon, shake dry, pluck off the leaves and chop. Arrange the roast turkey with the vegetables. Sprinkle tarragon on top.

This recipe is healthy because...

The summery light roast is wonderful for a figure-accentuating diet and you can indulge in aromatic vegetables. The colourful mixture guarantees a rich supply of micronutrients - for example niacin, zinc, vitamin C and biotin.

Nutritional values

1 Portion contains	(percentage of daily	requirement)
Calories	433 kcal	(21 %)
Protein	64 g	(65 %)
Fat	13 g	(11 %)
Carbohydrates	12 g	(8 %)
added sugar	0 g	(0 %)
Fibres	6 g	(8 %)

Day 7 Evening meal

Roast beef and beans salad with pumpkin seeds

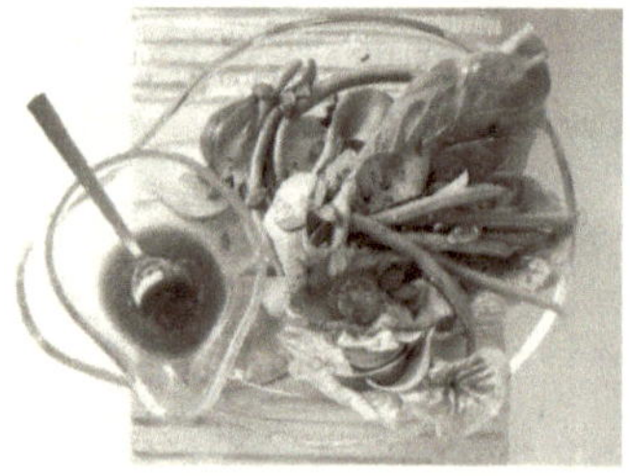

With this delicious dinner the low-carb week ends: roast beef bean salad with pumpkin seeds (354 calories per serving). This light dish contains protein, B vitamins and iron. The pumpkin seeds make the salad fun to nibble on and a good portion of vitamin E.

Difficulty: easy
Preparation: 35 Minutes
Calories: 354 Kcal

Ingredients for - 4 + portions

500 g string beans
Salt
100 g red onions (2 red onions)
300 g cherry tomatoes
6 savory stems
175 g Rocket salad (1 rocket salad)
4 tablespoon cider vinegar
3 tablespoon naturally cloudy apple juice
Pepper
4 tablespoon rape oil
2 tablespoon pumpkin seed oil
300 g roast beef cold cuts (in thin slices)
30 g pumpkin seeds

Preparation

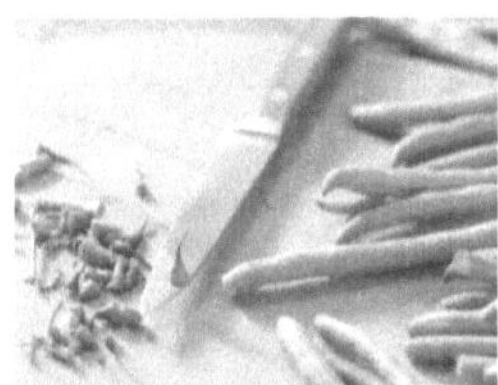

Wash and clean the beans and cook in boiling salted water for 10 to 12 minutes.

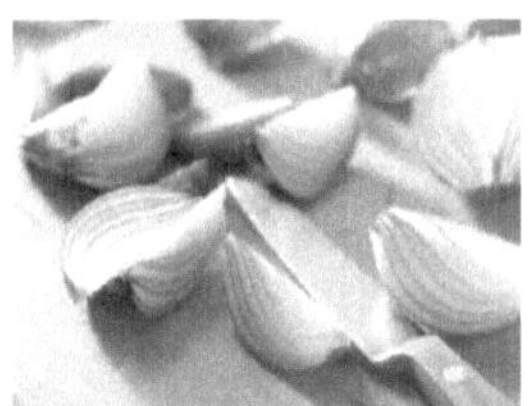

In the meantime peel the onions and cut them into 1 cm wide slices.

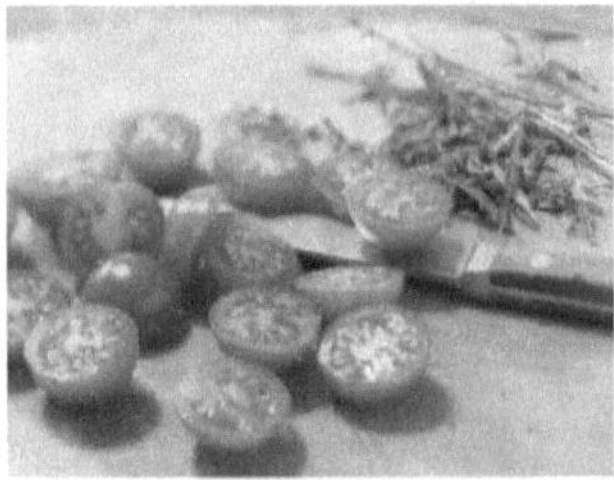

Wash the tomatoes, drain and cut in half. Wash the savory, shake dry, pluck off the leaves and chop roughly with a large knife.

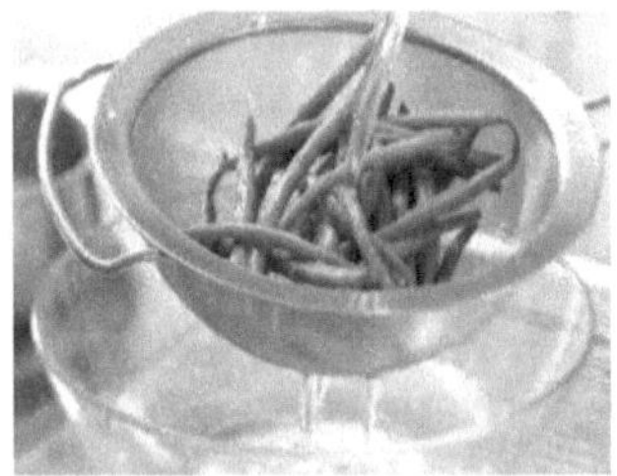

Drain the beans, rinse cold in a sieve and drain well.

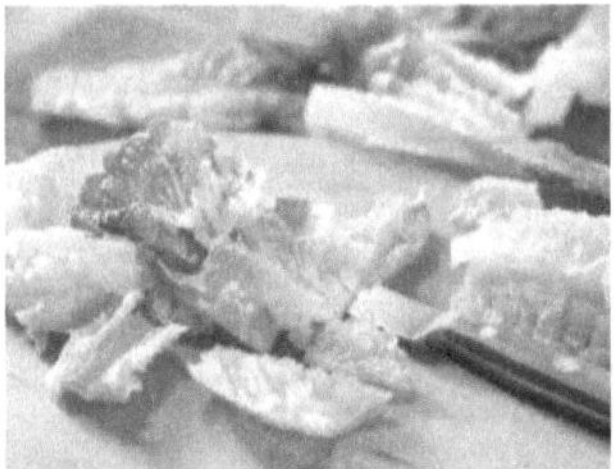

Clean, wash and spin-dry romaine lettuce and cut the leaves into bite-sized pieces.

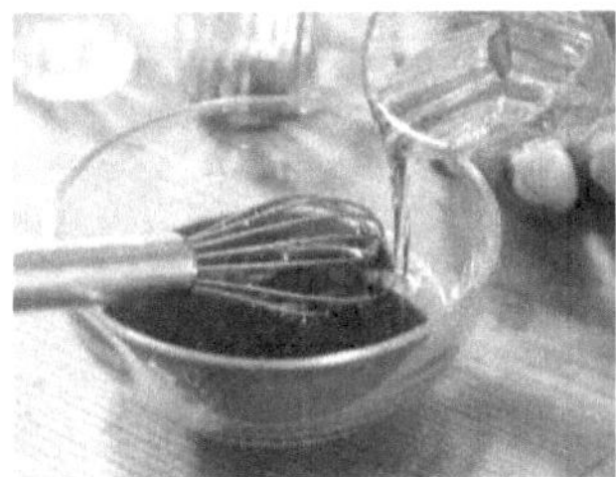

Mix vinegar in a small bowl with apple juice, salt and pepper. Stir in rapeseed and pumpkin seed oil bit by bit with a whisk and mix to a dressing.

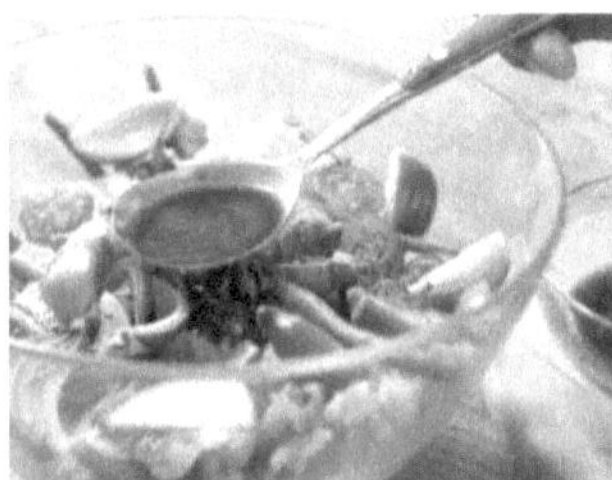

Place the savory with the beans, lettuce leaves, onions and tomatoes in a salad bowl. Mix in about 2/3 of the dressing.

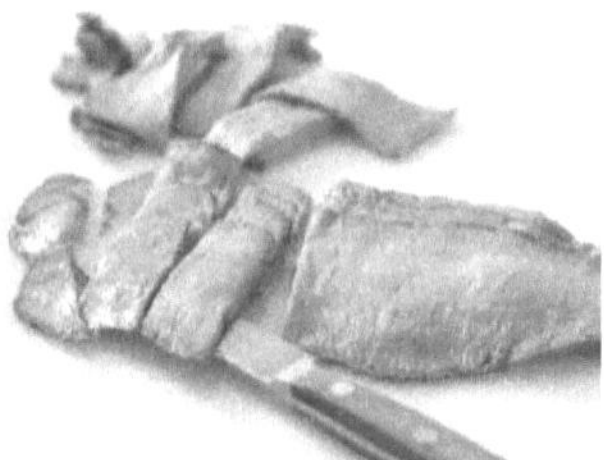

Cut roast beef slices into wide strips and carefully fold them into the bean salad. Season with salt and pepper, sprinkle with remaining dressing and sprinkle with pumpkin seeds.

This recipe is healthy because...

Beef and beans - always a nice pair! Especially when they present
themselves as finely as here and bring so much good with them.
Such as there are, for example: Protein, iron, nerve-strengthening
B vitamins and - thanks to the pumpkin seeds - the radical
scavenger vitamin E.

Nutritional values

1 Portion contains	(percentage of daily	requirement)
Calories	354 kcal	(17 %)
Protein	29 g	(30 %)
Fat	21 g	(18 %)
Carbohydrates	9 g	(6 %)
added sugar	0 g	(0 %)
Fibres	6 g	20 %)

Thank you very much for choosing my low-carb recipe book for a week. After reviewing it, please give me a review with the content of what you liked and / or did not like. Your review is very important to me to make my following books more sophisticated for you. I thank you in advance for taking the time for your review.